The Sir Jason Winters Story
Killing Cancer

BY
BENJAMIN ROTH SMYTHE
&
SIR JASON WINTERS

One hundred and fiftieth printing - 2009 USA
ISBN No. 1-885026-11-0

Published by
VINTON PUBLISHING CO.
PO Box 94075
Las Vegas, Nevada 89193

www.sirjasonwinters.com

A Message from Raymond Winters

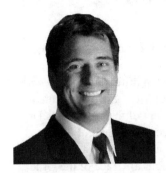

My Dear Friends,

Thank you for taking the time to read this book written by my father, Sir Jason Winters, along with Benjamin Roth Smythe. When it came time to reprint this book, I had the option of making changes. However, I decided to keep the book as it was written by my father. It is, after all, the story of his life, written in his own words. I have however changed the title as my father always wanted it to be "The Sir Jason Winters Story".

I want you to keep in mind as you read this book, it is for informational purposes only. Some information gathered and used by Sir Jason Winters when he wrote it may be outdated as it was written in the late 70's and first published in 1980.

My father tried many different things when he was ill and this book is not meant to be a guide for anyone to follow in attempt to heal an illness. If you are ill, please do your own research and see your doctor. As Sir Jason always said, you must seek the advice of a qualified health professional for all your health concerns.

Thank you for taking the time to read my father's story. It is my honor to share it with you.

My Very Warmest Regards,

Sir Raymond Winters
KCSJ SOJ

Sir Jason Winters' astounding worldwide success surprises the medical field, governments and natural health advocates.

- Over 13 million books in print.
- His products are available in over 70 countries and trusted by people worldwide.
- Sir Jason has won awards from seven different foreign governments, received an Award of Merit from the United States Congress, is two time recipient of the prestigious Dr. Albert Schweitzer Award, was given the Medal of Honor in Madrid, made Laureate of Belgium, Holland and South Africa, knighted in Malta as a Knight of Grace of the Order of St. John, to which Her Majesty the Queen and the Pope belong.
- Became the president of the World Federation of Integrated Medicine, formed in consultation with HRH Prince Charles.
- His formulas have been mentioned by dozens of authors and featured in over 100 health magazines worldwide.
- Seen on national television and heard on radio's Voice of America, BBC TV in London, Bombay Radio, Philippine TV and radio and newspapers around the world.
- Famous author Ruth Montgomery devoted an entire chapter to Jason Winters in her top selling book, *Threshold to Tomorrow*.
- Sir Jason does not believe that herbs cure any illness, but he has been assured by many herbalists that they do "strengthen the body and then the body can help itself." This is referred to in the Bible, and by Buddha, Krishna and Hippocrates. This is why 150 of the top prescription medicines come from herbs. Medical prescriptions written by doctors every day in America and England as well as many other countries contain herbs.
- Sir Jason Winter's objective is to get all of the healing arts, both orthodox and alternative, to work together for the benefit of mankind.
- For additional information about Sir Jason Winters, please visit his website at: www.sirjasonwinters.com

A PERSONAL LETTER FROM
SIR JASON WINTERS

I want to thank you for reading this book. Because of people like you, the world is changing. It has become obvious to all of us that medical science alone cannot solve all of our modern day maladies. Ancient remedies will not replace modern medical breakthroughs, but, as we are finding out quickly, they can certainly help tremendously. Ancient and natural therapies have been tried out over the centuries and the ones found to be effective are still in use today. Seventy-five years ago in England, for example, my grandmother, "Grandma Lewis" was busy helping distressed people by giving them St. John's Wort. Now, millions know that this herb works every bit as good as the modern day Prozac, with one big difference however—St. Johns Wort does not have any side effects and no withdrawal symptoms.

In 1920, Grandma Lewis was giving a mixture of garlic, gensing and ginger to the survivors of World War I who were suffering from shell shock, depression and shattered nerves. Her close relative, Lord Lewis, was on her health herbal formulas every day while serving in the British Parliament.

So, now you and I are aware that all healing arts must work together for the benefit of all. There can no longer be bitterness and hatred between orthodox and alternative practitioners. The time has come for open minds, more understanding and more compassion for all.

Since 1977, when I should have died, some very important people have helped me and I would be remiss not to thank them.

To Prince Charles, who placed his hand on my shoulder and said, "Don't worry, Mr. Winters, only God can tell you when you will die."

To the Archbishop of Canterbury, who, with Christian love, took time from his busy schedule to research the herb referred to so many times in the Bible.

To Dr. Ian Pierce who tested the herbal tea formula in the laboratory.

To Dr Malcolm Rae, who gave me such courage and strength.

To U.S. Congressmen James Bilbray and John Ensign for the award they gave me.

Thanks to Health Minister Hashimoto of Japan, Jaime Licoaco of the Philippines, and to Josef de Ubaldo of Manila, head of the Herbalist Association.

To Ruth Montgomery, America's favorite author, and finally, to the United States Surgeon General, for his invaluable report on antioxidants.

The author wishes to make it clear that he does not recommend total rejection of orthodox methods of treating illness, or a doctor's advice. If you are ill, see your doctor and tell him that you will do whatever he feels that you should. Then ask him if its all right if you change your diet to a more sensible one, and if he minds if you take herbs or herbal combinations. Any thinking doctor will see no problem with this.

Sir Jason Winters' objective is to get all of the healing arts, both orthodox and unorthodox, natural and chemical, to work together for the benefit of mankind.

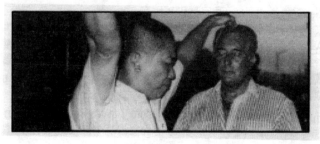

I tried everything to regain my health.

A Message From The Author

When I was first contacted by Jason Winters to write about his experiences I was very busy with other writings, and even though he was calling from the USA, I tried to put him off. He was quite persistent however, and finally I told him to send me the manuscript for my perusal. Within a week a package arrived and it consisted of cassette tapes, entitled "The Jason Winters Story". I listened to them with complete disinterest, then sat up and started to take notice. Something in this man's voice portrayed sincerity and great compassion.

His claims about cancer, herbs, laetrile, world travel and ultimate health, if true, were something the world should know about without delay.

First, I had to check out his story—the hospital, doctors, x-rays, cancer clinic, Dr. Malcolm Rae of Great Britain, and others. Then I started to check his sources of information, starting with the Bible, the writings of Buddha, Krishna, Bahá'u'lláh, and Hippocrates. Everything I found verifies Winters' story.

This took me six months, then I informed Winters that I would indeed write this little book for him. As always, I have written in the first person.

And so, dear reader, I give you *The Jason Winters Story*. May it be an inspiration to all who read it.

Benjamin Roth-Smythe

Author.

(Scientific Writer and Chemist)

TABLE OF CONTENTS

PREFACE

And God said, "Behold, I have given you every herb bearing seed which is upon the face of all the earth, and every tree in which is the fruit of a tree yielding seed: to you it shall be for meat." Gen 1:29

"And the fruit thereof shall be for meat, and the leaf thereof for medicine." Ezekiel 47:12

"He causeth the grass to grow for cattle, and herbs for the use of man." Psalm 104:14

"For one believeth he may eat all things; another who is weak eateth herbs." Romans 14:2

"And the leaves of the trees were for the healing of nations." Revelation 22:2

But powerful man-made organizations today tell us: What does God know? What does Buddha know? What does Hippocrates know? Take Aspirin, Bufferin, Valium and after the side effects of these have caused worse problems, have chemotherapy. When your hair falls out, buy a wig. I will give you prescriptions to deaden the pain, allow you to go through life like a zombie, and when you are too sick for us to help you anymore, then go home and prepare to die. But if you should obtain help from a herbalist, nutritionist, or any other than a doctor of medicine, then we will persecute him, if he makes you well, and prosecute him, if you should die as the original doctor said you would.

If you live, then we will laugh at you and harass you, and tell you that you were never ill in the first place.

I believe that if Jesus were to suddenly appear in America today to heal people, He would be arrested for practicing medicine without a license. Telling people that they can be healed by proper eating, thinking and living would result in an immediate jail sentence. They would not make Him walk the streets this time carrying a cross, but would rather crucify Him in all the establishment newspapers and other media. They would harass and ridicule Him, and they would drive Him out of the country.

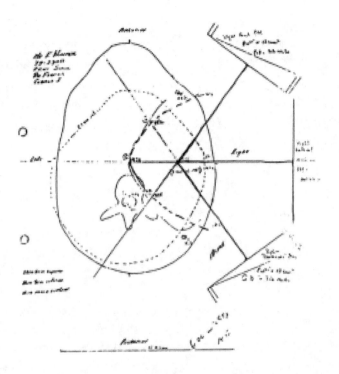

This is a medical drawing of Jason Winters' head based on actual X-ray photos. The view is from the top of the skull looking down. The shaded area marks the tumor.

Chapter 1

TERMINAL CANCER

I walked into the Cobalt Radiation Department for the first time and was filled with despair. This department took care of patients suffering from head and neck cancer. There were about 20 patients in the waiting room, and I took my place among them. My heart was thumping, and with good reason, for the faces all around me showed fear and depression. I could smell death in the air. Most of the people had hardly any hair left, due to the chemotherapy treatment. Ashtrays were scattered around the room and nearly everyone was smoking heavily. When I mentioned that smoking is bad for health, one patient said, "Well, it's too late for us now anyway, isn't it?"

One by one patients had their names called and they would disappear behind a large lead door. When they came out they looked worse than before—and left hurriedly. I was worried as I had no idea what was behind that door. Would I, too, soon have no hair and that look of terror in my eyes? I heard the nurse call my name, and as if in a daze, found myself following her into the treatment room.

I had first noticed the swelling on the side of my neck when taking a steam bath at the YMCA. Although 46 years old I was in top physical condition—running and swimming each day. I had a great wife, five kids and a good income. I smoked 30 cigarettes a day and did some real hard drinking at least once a week. Rye whiskey was my favorite.

The lump seemed to ache deep inside my throat. I was worried. I bought some lozenges and tried to forget about it. As the days went by the lump got bigger and bigger, but I avoided my doctor like the plague. I was unconsciously scared of what the lump might be. After a few more weeks even my friends noticed the swelling and remarked on it. I realized that I could not avoid the issue indefinitely, so I made an appointment with our family doctor.

He at once sent me to a surgeon. It resulted in dozens of x-rays, examinations at the Nuclear Medicine Center, scans, pills—and fear. At last it was decided that I must go into the hospital to have a small biopsy operation. The surgeon said it would take only half an hour and result in a scar a couple of inches long.

Soon after I checked into the hospital a dear old lady came around with lots of strong black coffee, white sugar and cream cake. She was trying hard to serve humanity and no one ever told her she was serving what I later found out to be the very worst things a cancer patient, or anyone else for that matter, can eat and drink.

I was scared to death, especially when they placed the mask over my face and I felt myself drifting away in a wave of terror.

Suddenly, everything was black, like the darkest night. I could see nothing, but for the first time in months I realized that I was not afraid; the air was cool and I breathed deeply and with every breath I felt stronger. Soon I saw a dim light far away so I started to drift towards it. I was walking but could not feel my legs or feet. It was effortless.

Soon I realized that I was in some kind of tunnel. Once I reached the entrance I noticed that I was wearing a long brown robe and pointed slippers that were covered in white dust.

Leaving the tunnel I was shocked by the sky. Words cannot explain how brilliantly blue it was. The pathway I had to walk was along the very peak of a line of mountains. The pathway was only six inches wide. There was a sheer drop on either side of the path, a drop that looked hundreds of feet deep. However, I could not see the bottom because there were dark clouds covering the ground far below me. From the depths of these clouds came the worst screams and moans that I had ever heard. Moans of total and complete despair. Moans I will never forget.

I had to walk carefully, or I would fall into the clouds below, and those terrible noises.

2

Suddenly the most brilliant of lights, so bright I could not look at it, was rushing down the path towards me. I could not move to either side to avoid it, so I crouched down and put up my arms for protection. The light passed right through me, and then I heard the nurse shouting, "More anesthetic quickly! He is regaining consciousness."

When I awoke from the operation I found that it had taken six and a half hours, and left a scar nine inches long. I saw immediately that my wife had been crying. I guess that was when I first knew for sure my condition was serious. The doctor walked in and said, "Terminal cancer. Infiltrating squamous cell carcinoma." The tumor was wrapped around my carotid artery and, to make matters even worse, was attached to the wall of my jugular vein.

After telling me three times that my condition was terminal, the doctor left me to my misery. My wife Jan went home to break the news to our five children. Thoughts of death crowded in on me from all sides. Reading, television, and radio were all drowned out by the thoughts that soon I would be gone.

The next morning, when my doctor made his rounds, he did not find me in bed. Another patient and I were having a hilarious pillow fight from our wheelchairs. The doctor was furious. "Don't you know you have terminal cancer? Don't you realize you should be in bed?" Because I was sure that all doctors are gods, I obeyed him quickly. It was not long before I was out of bed again—this time to trudge around the hospital.

I walked around the whole place five times for exercise, and when I returned it was the head nurse's turn to be furious. She said the doctor had been complaining to her about me, and once again assured me that I had terminal cancer, and must at least stay in my room.

It seemed to me that everyone was worried in case I forgot to die. The doctor even went so far as to lecture my wife on my behavior. "Doesn't he know he's got terminal cancer? Doesn't he believe me?"

Many tests followed and finally it was agreed what my treatment should be. I would have five weeks of cobalt radiation on my neck and head, and then if the swelling were down, I could have radical neck surgery. That meant the removal of my tongue, jaw bone, neck muscles, and also the inside of my throat. To begin with I would receive three cobalt treatments each day for five weeks.

I felt better as soon as I left the hospital and walked down the street. I felt free, even though I got a lot of stares from people gaping at the bandages around my face and neck. At least they couldn't see the tumor.

My first appointment with the cancer clinic bothered me. I had to be fitted for a plastic mask. This went right over my head like the Count of Monte Cristo mask. There were three holes in one side for it to be attached to the cobalt machine, so that I could not move my head while being bombarded with radiation. I had to go back in one week for another fitting, and this really depressed me. I got so bad that I would not let my wife tell anyone that I had cancer. I could not stand the look of fear in their faces and the way even old friends changed towards me. I would not even let my children say the word cancer.

The nurse in the cobalt room called my name—and it started.

For five weeks I was to see my fellow patients gradually get weaker and weaker—then I would see them no more. One friend was a big strong man and had a tumor on the side of his head. After many cobalt treatments his right eye started running, so they sewed it closed. I will always remember the terror in his one good eye, as he looked at me in desperation. I said, "Don't worry, we will both get better," not believing it myself of course.

My friend beamed and he shouted to all the other patients. "Did you hear that? Jason says we are both going to get better!" It was many months later that I understood what he meant and why he was so happy. Since he had discovered he had cancer, he had been told repeatedly, "Terminal, terminal." I was the first one in the whole wide world to tell him he would get better, or to offer even any hope at all. He died two days later. I started taking Valium tablets each day so that I would not break down and cry, as well as pain pills and sleeping pills.

The cobalt treatment took away my taste, made it impossible for me to make saliva, burned the right side of my face and made my hair fall out. Life was hell.

I went from 263 lb. down to 170 lb. My knees were shaky and I could not stay awake for longer than four hours at a time. It was then that I discovered the value of pure honey and vitamin E. As I would sit on the couch in shock, after the cobalt treatment, I would eat spoonfuls of honey which I could not taste but I knew was good for me. I stopped losing weight. I smeared the vitamin E on my burned face, and soon there was a great improvement. Doctors at the cancer clinic remarked how well I was taking the treatment. I told them what I was doing and they said that this was fine, but I was not to mention it to the others.

That remark puzzled me no end. I thought about it constantly. I did tell the others about it and they all started the same treatment with good results. But the doctors did not want me to tell anyone about it. The only answer I could figure out to this scared the heck out of me, but it probably saved my life. I started to realize that doctors are not gods after all. Maybe they can make mistakes too. If that was right, then maybe they had made a mistake about me. They all kept telling me to get my affairs in order, and prepare to die, but perhaps I didn't have to die.

The next day the surgeon called me into his office. He had decided to operate on me as soon as possible. Radical neck surgery. Removal of tongue, jaw bone and neck muscles. He went into great detail about the operation. When I asked him if I would live any longer from having the surgery, he said probably not. I looked him straight in the eye and said, "No."

5

The doctor said, "What do you mean, no?"

I said, "No operation." Then I stood up and walked out of his office. My heart was singing. I was going to keep my tongue and die in one piece.

Many times the doctor called my wife to tell her to get me into the hospital. Everyone was trying to get me there, even though they knew that I would die anyway. I couldn't understand it. I wondered who these people thought they were, asking me to have this terrible operation.

Then I heard about Laetrile.

Chapter 2

Laetrile

I heard that Laetrile was made from apricot kernels and contained a little cyanide, necessary in our body in small amounts. I went at once to the health food store and bought six bottles of apricot kernels. I would eat about 50 a day. Soon the aching stopped and it looked as though the tumor was actually shrinking. I was elated and overjoyed. I did not worry about being cured. Just as long as I could keep it under control would be good enough for me.

When I ran out of the kernels I returned to the health food store for more. I was told that the government authorities had removed them from the shelves. I was horrified. How could anyone do this? The man in the health food store offered a possible explanation. Laetrile may control cancer without all the operations and radiation that I had been through. What would happen to those people who work in cancer clinics by the thousands? They would be unemployed of course. Drug companies would lose millions, as would doctors, surgeons, anesthetists and nurses. Thirty major countries of the world use Laetrile in the treatment of cancer, but in North America it was banned.

Now I had not yet got over the fact that doctors could make mistakes, so it took a lot of thought and investigation before I could realize the monstrous evil behind banning apricot kernels and Laetrile. Dying people are sent home with the words, "We can't do anything for you," without the right even to try possibly the biggest natural cancer fighter of all time.

I heard that the Contreras Clinic in Tijuana, Mexico, gave Laetrile to patients, and my heart leapt. My wife and family made arrangements to accompany me, and off we went to Mexico.

We arrived at Centro Medico Del Mar in Tijuana early in the morning, and were soon surrounded by hundreds of Americans

7

and Canadians, all in the same position as myself. However there was a difference from the other cancer clinics, for here I could see hope and enthusiasm shining on everyone's face. After a complete examination by a doctor I was scheduled for Laetrile injections each day and also put on a diet. I felt better already. For the first time in my life I started eating sensibly. Part of the treatment must be correct diet. Slowly I started building up my body. I thought of the old lady at the hospital with her coffee, white sugar and cream buns—all definite taboos at the clinic. Almost everyone here had a miraculous story to tell. I was slowly emerging from that long black tunnel of death, and I was ecstatic.

All of the patients here were terminal patients from the U.S. and Canada who had exhausted every avenue or orthodox treatment and now were trying this as a last resort. But miracles were happening here, and I thanked God that I had heard about it.

Each morning I would join in the line with hundreds of patients and when my turn came I would go into a cubicle and receive an enzyme enema. Right after this would come the Laetrile injection. I can honestly say that there were no adverse effects experienced either by myself or any of the others. In ten days the tumor had shrunk to half the size and the doctor stated that I could return home, but must take some Laetrile tablets with me. I should take these three times each day. He said that my cancer was under control. I emerged from the clinic a happy man, hardly able to believe my good fortune.

When I arrived home I found that the cancer clinic had called many times. They wanted me to go up in front of a panel of doctors to be examined. They were all sure that I would have to have the operation. They knew nothing of my trip to Mexico.

I arrived early for the examination, eager to see the expression on their faces when they discovered the tumor almost gone. One by one they examined me. But not one of them said a word to me. There were no smiles, no congratulations, no happiness at all. When I finally told them I had been taking Laetrile, the doctor who had wanted to remove my tongue said that I could not have had cancer in the first place. Another said he must perform the operation anyway. I was horrified at the way these people acted, and left as soon as possible.

I thought the doctors would be overjoyed that my tumor had gone, and would demand to know how I had done it, then hold press conferences around the world, stating just what had happened. I thought of the thousands who were waiting for cobalt treatment, or were swallowing chemotherapy poison, so bad for the system it makes the patients' hair fall out, makes them vomit continuously and fills the body full of toxins. I thought of the thousands who were waiting to enter the operating rooms of hospitals around the country, waiting to have tumors removed or colostomies. Terrible operations that removed the effects but not the cause. I thought of all the thousands who that very week would be told they had cancer, and of how they would start dying immediately because to them just the word *cancer* meant certain death. I felt like running through every cancer clinic in North America shouting that there is possibly a control for cancer. Don't let that little old lady fill your ailing bodies with poisonous coffee and white sugar. Start eating God's health foods right now.

Chapter 3

NUTRITION

Now I know for sure that some readers are just as naive as I was about cancer, the medical profession, Laetrile and all alternative therapies. I know that some people are so stubborn that they would die rather than admit they are wrong—and often do. If it's only your own life at stake, do as you wish, but if you are concerned with someone else's life, such as a loved one, a friend or relative, then remember, you are not God, and they deserve the benefit of the doubt. The whole reason for this book is to make you doubt. Then maybe you will search for the truth.

"Things that are sweet in the mouth are bitter in the stomach." We know that too much sugar and sweet things are bad for us. And things that are bitter in the mouth are sweet in the stomach. Bitter almonds and apricot kernels are very bitter, and this is what Laetrile is made from. God wants us to be healthy, so he gave us everything we need to live long healthy lives. In this age of people proudly stating, "My son, the doctor," I fear that we have made doctors our gods. It is interesting to note that in Oden's book, *Thank God I have Cancer*, it is shown that doctors and their families are among the unhealthiest in the nation. I quote:

10% already have cancer.

12% already have anemia.

21% have allergies.

24% have had major surgery.

30% are overweight.

These are the people that we run to with our sick bodies. These are the people we run to, instead of God. By the thousands we rush to psychiatrists, asking them to straighten out our minds. In reality psychiatrists have the highest suicide rate of any group in the world. These are facts. Once in a while it is possible to find a doctor who works with nature and with God. This person will rely mainly on natural foods, vitamins and minerals to help your body regain health. Find a doctor who believes God is greater than the medical associations, and you have found a jewel.

He will suggest you eat properly and he may well recommend B17 (Laetrile) because he will be unbiased and really care about you. He makes no money from Laetrile, and there is no drug salesman giving him free samples. This man cares so much because God is his boss—not a medical association. I feel that medical associations are like unions: designed to keep their members busy and financially secure. Can you name a nation other than America where a doctor expects to make hundreds of thousands of dollars each year? Can you name another country where doctors will not make house calls? Where they expect to retire at such an early age? Where they will charge you for not showing up for an appointment, but can keep you waiting for hours? Do they make money from sickness, or health? Supposing that eating properly, along with God's natural immunity that He has given us all, kept everyone healthy, what would happen to the biggest business in America today?

It is interesting to note that in some provinces of China a doctor is paid, by the government, a flat fee each month. When anyone gets sick, the doctor is fined a small amount. You see, he failed to keep his people healthy. He makes money out of health, whereas our doctors only can survive if we keep getting ill.

Find a God-loving, nutritionally conscious doctor and you may avoid the treadmill of death. That is what I call orthodox cancer treatment. First the radiation which burns and sears, then the operation which removes the effect and not the cause, which also leaves you weak and in shock, and finally, if you have survived this, you are given chemotherapy. You are ill because your body is full of poisons, but now they are pouring more down your throat. Poison so drastic that sometimes they have to stop the treatment for a while so you can get stronger. Imagine a medicine so toxic that they have to take you off it so that you will get stronger by yourself. You have suffered all of this and yet God's system is still working within you. But oh, how it needs help. Nutrition. A change of mind about cancer, the treadmill of death. If you are an American, from the time you are told you have cancer until you die, you will have spent an average of seventy thousand dollars. A doctor told me that once he or his associates discover cancer in a patient, they mentally write him off. He is as good as dead. I think doctors convey this attitude of helplessness to the patient.

Now I am a firm believer in mind over matter. So that if you have made a god of your doctor, then you will certainly do what he tells you, even to the extent of dying as expected. After all, faith can move mountains. Then why shouldn't you die when your medical god tells you that you should? It is hard to change from a negative to a positive attitude, especially when you have been bombarded with radiation, cut up with surgery and then poisoned with chemotherapy. But talk to the thousands of people at the Laetrile clinics in Mexico and Germany. They all go to these clinics after the medical profession has given up on them. My telling you what is taking place there every day is not enough. You must take full responsibility for your own life. You must find out this exciting truth for yourself.

Some people of course are so stubborn that they cannot be helped. Although it is heartbreaking there is nothing you can do. The following story is a typical example.

Two young boys, one ten years old and one seven had tumors in the legs. The seven-year-old's parents were well aware of nutritional cures. When told that major surgery was necessary they refused, and the boy was put on a nutritional diet and Laetrile. Six weeks later the tumor was gone and he has complete remission. His smiling, happy face is a glorious sight to behold.

However, the ten-year-old's parents believed that if there was another treatment for cancer then the doctors would know about it. When they asked their doctor about Laetrile he called it a useless toxic hoax, used by charlatans and quacks.

As of this writing the little boy is waiting for his third operation. He has already lost his left leg. His hair has fallen out. My heart goes out to him and to the thousands of others on his medically approved treadmill of death.

Can you imagine what would happen if suddenly the truth were to come out? As Red Buttons, the comedian, said to reporters of the National Inquirer, "People who suppress Laetrile and stop other people from using it are nothing more than murderers." Buttons' wife gained remission of cancer through Laetrile.

Fred McMurray of TV fame gained remission of cancer through Laetrile. A wonderful man who said "No" to orthodox methods and took the natural way back to health.

People involved in Laetrile have been persecuted. Many have been to court and won the case, only to be taken to court again and again. This is harassment. Even though a person wins every case, he can go broke just defending himself. So the million-dollar drug cartels win after all. One top doctor told me that as long as more people benefit from cancer than suffer from it, we will be happy to go along just like this. Hundreds of millions are spent on cancer research each year, providing many top-paying jobs. A startling fact to remember in all of this is that statistics indicate that one person in four will have cancer next year. No wonder, the way we are eating and drinking junk. No wonder our bodies are fighting a losing battle.

In spite of all the persecutions and harassments, those pushing for the right of patients to use Laetrile are winning. We can now obtain Laetrile (B17 or amygdalin) in most states and provinces although it's not easy and it is expensive. It is estimated that three thousand people in Canada alone order Laetrile every month. They have to order it from Germany or Mexico because the homemade stuff is not always pure. The average person spends about one hundred dollars each month on Laetrile, which means that over three hundred thousand dollars each month are leaving a country with a population of just twenty million.

To get an idea of how much Americans are spending on Laetrile each month, just multiply that figure by ten. Laetrile is a God-given vitamin that attacks cancer cells and is completely nontoxic if obtained in its pure form.

The largest manufacturer of Laetrile in Europe ships out over five hundred thousand orders each month to doctors, hospitals, clinics and patients all over the world. Also, Laetrile in the form of bitter almonds and apricot kernels has been in use to fight tumors for 4000 years. Recently, while browsing through a book store in London, I was surprised to come across a book, first published in 1810 and written by Jacob Antworth. On page 81 he states that in order to eliminate growths, the kernels from apricots should be crushed and mixed with your morning oats! You will be glad to know that God did not put all His eggs in one basket, so to speak. The following foods all contain Laetrile: alfalfa, buckwheat, cassava, flaxseed, broad beans, lima beans, garlic, soya beans, berries, blackstrap molasses, macadamia nuts, sprouts, rye, rice, bran, peas, oats, millet and the seeds of apple, plum, cherry and of course apricot. So start helping yourselves to God's way of killing cancer. Pancreatic enzymes are also very important to the cancer patient. Two tablets taken prior to Laetrile allow the latter to work more effectively. It seems that the enzymes rush to the cancerous area where they start eating away at the protein shell that usually surrounds and protects a tumor. This allows the Laetrile to penetrate the tumor and release its cyanide onto the cancer cells to kill them.

When you remember that all natural means were given to us by God, it means that the authorities have rejected God's methods.

Americans told by their doctors to prepare to die are filling clinics in Mexico and Germany and many are going home in a few weeks with their cancer in complete remission. These clinics are not run by quacks either. Most of the world's foremost cancer scientists believe that Laetrile is a wonderful anticancer agent.

Among them are Dr. N. R. Boujiane in Montreal, Dr. John Morrone in New Jersey, Dr. Hans Nieper in Germany, Dr. Contreras in

Mexico and Dr. Navarro in Manila. Of course the findings of such men are discounted in America. They dare to take a different stand, and so are often ridiculed. Jesus was persecuted for being different, and Giordano Bruno was burned at the stake for teaching that the world is round. Laetrile works in many, many cases and is certainly worth a try. It takes away the pain and makes one far more comfortable.

I have spoken to hundreds of people who should have died twenty years ago, according to their doctors, but they discovered Laetrile and have taken it daily ever since and are as healthy as can be. I have gone into the Laetrile story at great lengths because I am about to shock you, and before I do I want you to know that Laetrile works for thousands of people.

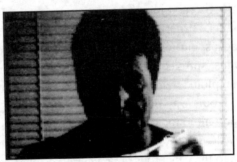

1977 - Sir Jason Winters
Undergoing Cobalt Radiation Treatment.

My tumor started coming back. I was taking the enzymes and the three thousand milligrams of Laetrile every day, but the swelling started coming back. In shock, I increased the dosage but it did no good whatsoever.

After three weeks the tumor was as big as it was before, so I called the Laetrile clinic. I was told that this sometimes but rarely happens, and there was not much that I could do. I was on a strict diet of fruit and vegetables with large doses of vitamins, but it was getting worse.

Now I really did live with death 24 hours each day. It was as though I had been given life, only to have it snatched away. This time I really did prepare to die. I purchased all kinds of religious books and while my family went to work to keep groceries on the table, I read them all. In my misery I was struck by how many times herbs are mentioned in the Bible, even on the first page. Herbs as medicines show up in so many different religions that it seemed to be too much of a coincidence. Hippocrates, father of medicine, stated that herbs shall be for medicine. So did Buddha and Krishna. Then I found that the North American Indians believed in herbs and used them as medicine; also the Gypsies of Europe, and the Hunzas, and the Aborigines. All spiritual writings somewhere or other mention herbs for healing.

In desperation my mind cast about to decide what I should do. It would be so easy to do nothing, and to waste away. I was full of dread and fatigue. But I could not die yet. Besides, I was too scared to die. I must find the herbs that God put here for this purpose. And so started a search around the world.

Chapter 4

HEALING HERBS

Once I started learning about herbs as medicine I became excited, especially after my letdown with Laetrile. The most powerful ancient herb for tumors seemed to come from Asia. I went to every herbalist in my area, then telephoned others across the country. They had never heard of it except in old books from Asia. The more difficult this herb became for me to find the more determined I was to have it. BUDDHA CALLED IT HERBALENE.

When I learned that it was available in Singapore, I started thinking about travelling there. The only problem was money. We had six thousand dollars to our name, did not own a house or anything else worthwhile that I could get a loan on. Also we had five kids to support. But still, we all felt that this was a matter of life and death. My eldest child went to stay with friends, and my sixteen- and fifteen-year-old sons quit school (we hoped, temporarily) and got jobs. I had many credit cards left over from my more affluent days and I figured I would use these to pay travel expenses. If I survived, then I would pay them back, and if not, my wife would have to declare bankruptcy. So it came about that with our two youngest children, my wife and I boarded a plane—destination Singapore. The fact that my two children had to support me, one under each arm, caused the Singapore immigration some concern. For a moment it was touch and go on whether they would let me into the country. We explained that I was merely airsick, which I am sure they did not believe, as the tumor was obvious to all. They decided in our favor and we soon found ourselves at the hotel. I lost no time in looking for the herb, which was not available in the stores in Singapore. At last I came upon an old lady living a distance from town, who cultivated the herb.

Evidently she dug up the roots and boiled 50 lb. in a large container. After boiling vigorously for twenty-six hours, she was left with a liquid concentrate which she sold for a very high price.

19

Usually sold in half-ounce bottles, she was surprised when I asked for one pint. I was told it would definitely get rid of my cancer. I can remember that I held that bottle with great reverence—after all, this is the very thing that the great Buddha suggested for tumors. I could hardly wait to get back to the hotel to start drinking it. The directions were to take one-eighth of a teaspoonful in a large glass of water, once each day, until well.

For ten days I took the medicine, and when nothing happened I doubled the dose. The tumor, although not getting any bigger stayed the same size exactly. A hurried visit to the old lady brought merely a shrug. She had no idea why it had not worked. She said, "Well, at least it's stopped growing," and that was it. My wife insisted that we buy another pint from her, even though we still had a lot left over. Jan was so impressed by the old lady's knowledge that she figured even if it did not cure cancer, it would prevent her getting it. Both her parents had died of the disease.

We left Singapore feeling very low indeed. I felt the herb did not work, and maybe that was why it didn't. We left for our next destination which was Tucson, Arizona.

Years before I had been a stunt man and a bit actor in Hollywood. We had made a few films with Audie Murphy in a place called Old Tucson, just a few miles from Tucson. Old Tucson was built in the Old West style for Hollywood. Many western movies were made there, including "Apache Agent," in which I played. I had learned at that time about a tea which most Indians, especially Mexican Indians, drank for health, and that's what prompted our visit. In Arizona we soon located the herb, known as chaparral, or the creosote bush (Larrea divaricata). Once again we heard that this remedy had been passed down through the ages and may prevent or get rid of cancer.

We stayed at the Santa Rita Hotel in Tucson, then moved to a small motel with a kitchen. The chaparral tea which I had to make five times each day was putrid, and smelled as bad as it tasted. It was enough to make a healthy man sick, but I persisted. It seemed to do nothing at all, except make me sick, but looking back now I feel that although I was not getting better, I was not getting worse. But at the time, so obsessed with death and dying, I was too depressed to notice.

In Tucson, a nutritionist who learned of my condition told us that in Europe there were many old remedies for different ills, even cancer. He said that because there is socialized medicine there (free doctors and hospitals), doctors don't expect to become rich overnight. Because of this they are more open to inexpensive alternative therapies. He said that if ever he became ill he would return to England for that reason alone. And so, as a last resort, we decided to visit England.

With five pounds of chaparral and a pint and a half of the Singapore potion we boarded the plane for London. We had already spent most of our cash and were now on credit cards. That was the only time in my life that I have ever appreciated credit. In one clinic I met HRH Prince Charles who gave me hope.

Now I have dozens of relatives in England, but I would not let my wife contact any of them. I did not want them to see me like this, and I wanted no tears. This is the part of the trip that I enjoyed, because this was the country I was born in, and it did me good to see the beautiful countryside once more. In my heart I knew that the visit was not really necessary, but just returning home meant defeat, and going to England postponed the inevitable for a while.

The Archbishop of Canterbury introduced me to red clover (Trifolium pratense), the Gypsy health drink that is supposed to be good for many things. Evidently there is a big difference between red and white clover blossoms, with the white being inferior. White clover is sold all over North America as being the best.

Chopped up clover blossoms make a very nice tea, which I started drinking, also at the rate of five glasses each day. This meant that I was busy making tea all day, first with the Asian herb, the chaparral, then red clover.

21

On the fourth day I became very ill indeed. My legs were shaking and I felt terribly sick. I had to stay in bed. I stopped taking all the herbs and readied myself for death. Our credit cards were promptly confiscated and we found we owed many thousands of dollars. Bill collectors were calling on the telephone and knocking on the door constantly; we were all very worried. My youngest son, Robin, was sent home from school because he broke down and started crying. When asked why he said, "My dad is dying of cancer."

As a last resort, I started back on the herbal teas again. One morning, I can remember it well, I was at my lowest ebb. I thought to heck with it, I'll mix all the herbs together.

Chapter 5

THE MIXTURE

It was five minutes to ten on a Wednesday morning. I made the tea combination and a miracle happened.

I could feel it with that first swallow. It seemed to ring a distant bell, a long-past memory. It screamed at me that this was what I needed. Strength seemed to pour through my body. That day I made a gallon of the tea and drank it all. When my family walked through the door they could see the difference in my face. I was enthusiastic, excited and overjoyed. Tears filled all of our eyes. We did not understand what had happened but we all knew that something wonderful had taken place. Day after day I drank one gallon regularly. Strength and vitality returned, but mostly it was my frame of mind. I was going to live, I knew it. All depression left me, all morbid thoughts. The more excited I became the smaller the tumor got; the smaller the tumor became, the more I got excited. Within three weeks the tumor had gone completely. Everyone called it a miracle, because in nine weeks I returned to work. I was not as healthy as before, I was healthier, and God, how I enjoyed every minute of life.

My case became well known throughout the news media and people with terminal cancer started lining up outside the door, just to talk to me. They all wanted the tea. Then my local priest called me into his office and said, "Look, Jason, I know, and so do you, that you have found something for good health. Why, my hemorrhoids, that I have suffered with for twenty years, disappeared in two weeks of drinking your tea. Many other things are happening to people drinking it too. Good things. You have something here, and if you do nothing about it you will be guilty of the sin of omission. But if you do decide to do something about it, you can expect to be persecuted severely. The officials won't let you ruin a multimillion-dollar-a-year business without a fight, and they have the money and the power to ridicule you, and to threaten you."

After much thought I decided to tell my story to the world. A small newspaper took up the story first, which resulted in over three hundred telephone calls and a thousand letters, plus a big line-up outside the door, from eight AM until past midnight. Everyone wanted the tea. Separately the herbs would not work for me; together they were a miracle. I started importing the ingredients and mixing them in five-ounce bags, which I would give to anyone who wanted some. In exchange they would give a donation so that I could get more herbs. Thank God for Dr. Ian Pearce, M.D., for explaining why the formula works.

The radio station told my story, which increased the customers tenfold. Never in the history of the radio station had they received so many calls as they did about that particular program.

One man with a brain tumor received such help that the doctors pronounced him well. Without my permission he had advertising made up about my tea. He wanted the world to know about it—he wanted to help everyone. He got me into trouble and my first persecutions began.

People started flying in to see me from Australia, Germany, and many other places in the world, and I was flooded under. The police became regular visitors to my place, making sure that I did not tell anyone that the herbs were any good for anything. But I didn't need to say anything. The world was so desperate for something natural that would work that I was constantly running out of herbs.

I started receiving many offers from people and companies, one even from a priest. I had never met this man before, but he came up to me and said, "Take me in as your partner and we will make a million. We can charge fifty dollars a four-ounce bag, and I can get the hell out of this church." All this, in front of a witness! I found it hard to believe, and told him a definite "No."

Now the priest had in his congregation a particularly violent man who needed help desperately. The priest, mad at me for not accepting his offer, set this man on me. He actually attacked me once in the church. The priest would incite the man, whom I will call Mr. H. Strangely enough, one of the first letters reporting benefits from the tea came from Mr. H.'s wife. So furious were the priest and Mr. H. that they typed letters to magazines and newspapers, and sometimes even to dying people, saying, "Mr. Winters never had cancer, and if you want more information call Reverend...," and of course the letters were unsigned. So persecution and hatred come from various places. When a national magazine ran a 28-page story on my experiences and the tea, they took three months to put it together, and interviewed hundreds of people involved.

As far as the editors are concerned the tea works, and now they are steady drinkers of it themselves. At the time the article was being prepared, the Canadian version of the FDA showed up and went through our files, taking the names of all our customers and confiscating all the tea we had. By this time I had three thousand people relying on me for the tea. They took up a collection and I left for Nassau in the Bahamas where I set up a company.

When the article came out in the magazine, we started receiving over 2000 orders each day, and that has continued with absolutely no advertising whatsoever. We had to hire all the unemployed people we could get to help us, and still the business grew. Over one thousand letters each month poured in telling of the relief obtained from all kinds of ills. Hollywood stars, politicians, all types of medical men, attorneys, truck drivers, order regularly.

Greed caused people to do some pretty terrible things—the priest previously mentioned, for instance. Knowing that I had left the country, he gathered a group of people around him and they are now selling an herbal mix using my name, knowing that it is nowhere near the same tea. A health food distribution company in Toronto also could see the money in this, and is putting out a phony tea under my name. These people are of course trading lives for dollars, and I mention this so that the reader knows enough to be careful. I have recently turned over the formula and all rights to a large manufacturer of herbal preparations. The hatred, bitterness, greed and harassment proved too much for me to handle. Besides this, my values have changed. Money is not as important to me as being alive. I feel wonderful about life, and about God, who cured me. Greed and bitterness cause stress, and I think that stress causes cancer, so I will leave all those feelings behind.

GOOD NEWS FROM SAUDI ARABIA
AND ENGLAND

People all over the world started drinking our tea, which has now become known as possibly the best health drink in the world. The only complaint we received, however was from people asking if the taste could be made a little less bitter.

It was in England where Dr. Ian Pierce, M.D., told me that one other herb was exchangeable for chaparral (the bitter one), and that was sage.

In the year 1620, a famous Arab physician claimed, "How can a man become ill, with this herb growing in the garden?" But I was to find out that there are over one hundred types of sage, some with health benefits and many without. I decided to find out for myself which herbal sage the Arabian doctor had been referring to. It was not as difficult a search as I had thought. Herbalists in the Middle East had used the same herb for centuries to treat people for every illness nnder the sun.

When I obtained some, mixed it with red clover and spice (I did this on my table in the kitchen) I was so pleased with the results that the same day I invited everyone that came to the house, including the mailman, the next door neighbors and the local policeman, to try it. They all thought it was delicious. Yet it still got the same results as the previous blend.

Here at last we had a good drink that tasted great. But still some diehards demanded the chaparral formula. And so, for many years we produced both. There really is no need to put up with a bitter taste any more and as an alternative to coffee, regular tea and soft drinks, this is the answer. The Japanese were the first ones to put this new Jason Winters Herbal Tea into soft drink cans, and people of all ages love it.

So, if you are worried about chaparral, don't be. It seems that God helps us every step of the way.

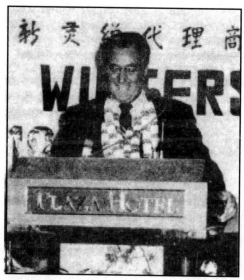

Live audience plus television and radio seminar in Malaysia.

Chapter 6

WHY THE HERB COMBINATION WORKS

God placed a certain herb on each continent to cure illness by simply purifying the blood. Life is in the blood, and if anything purifies the blood then a person's God-given natural immunity will have a chance to take over and fight all disease.

It is as simple as that.

The herb God put in Asia will not grow elsewhere, and the same goes for chaparral of North America and red clover of Europe. If you try to grow these herbs elsewhere they do not thrive because of soil deficiencies.

Jesus spoke of one herb for purifying the blood, Buddha of another herb in Asia, and the North American spirit fathers of yet another. Now in those days, before coffee, white sugar, processed foods and fast food outlets, any one of these herbs would have done the trick on its own. However, we alive today have such toxic bodies that we don't know what good health really is; after all we have nothing to judge it by. We are fed on canned milk from birth, then doctored up cow's milk, canned baby food, graduating to hamburgers, french fries, coffee and poisonous white sugar. That is why just one of these herbs would not work on me. I was so full of toxins, as are you, that it took the combined effort of three of the most powerful herbs to bring me back to health.

I did not know it at the time, but while I was drinking the tea, at first I became sick to my stomach. I should have noticed this as a good sign. All that was happening was that the herbs were clearing my body of poison, and it was taking place so fast that it was overpowering my liver. What a person should do in that case is take it easy for three days, then start on the herbs again. Eventually the body will be pure and you will not feel sick any more.

On a recent trip to England I was met with open arms by the medical profession. They were eager to try my tea. One radionics practitioner tested the tea with his machine and found that it raised his energy level from 47 to 88. This may not mean much to the average reader, but to anyone in the know about radionics it is quite astounding. We immediately got calls from reporters wanting interviews and these people were not the slightest bit hesitant about printing the facts about the tea. What a difference from America where the newspapers keep well away from anything like this, unless they are accusing you of something. Even the British royal family have their own herbalist, a Mrs. Blackie, who has treated the Queen and her family for years.

The highlight of my trip to England was meeting two wonderful men, Dr. Ian Pearce and Malcolm Rae. In Dr. Pearce we found a medical doctor with an open mind. I shall always remember sitting in his cottage in Norfolk, listening to him talk about herbs. Mr. Rae, on the other hand, was one of the world's leading radionics practitioners. Sadly he died at the end of 1979. He placed the tea on a machine and startled us by saying that the tea worked not only on the physical level, but also on the mental and spiritual planes. Why this startled me is that the old lady in Singapore had said, "This herb will bring the spiritual and mental bodies back into line with the physical body." At the time I did not understand it, but I did when Malcolm Rae explained it. It is simply a matter of treating the whole person, not just a particular illness. You must treat the mental, spiritual and physical before you can obtain perfect health.

Malcolm Rae then examined me by machine and found that although I had no cancer, I was suffering from cobalt radiation poisoning of the jaw bone, but that the tea was ridding me of that slowly.

Upon our arrival back in Nassau we found thousands of complaints from people who had not received their tea, ordered weeks before. We checked back and found that all had been sent via the Post Office within two days of receiving the order. It seemed as though the powers that be had finally found a way to stop us from helping people. During a period of three months over 10,000 packets of tea disappeared in the post, and we never have found them. The customers, knowing nothing of our problems, started to write some pretty awful letters to us, some even blaming us for their spouse's death.

This of course bothered me to no end, so we kept sending out second orders free, by the thousands. In spite of all our troubles, the letters kept coming in telling of health improvements in arthritis, varicose veins, hemorrhoids, skin problems and much more. Now that the herbs are supplied by one company these problems have been solved.

Along with complaints come pitiful, sad stories—some that have made us weep. One lady sent back the tea, saying, "My doctor says I have only a month or so to live and he doesn't want me using this stuff." And another, "My husband sneaks your tea into the hospital every night in a thermos. The doctor would be furious if he knew what it was but we told him it's brandy. He feels better each day and the doctor thinks it's his doing." But the saddest case of all is the following. A woman of 35 came to me because she had cancer of the breast. I spoke to her about my case and she became a different person, excited and happy. She visited her doctor that afternoon and he told her that the cancer had spread to her right eye and brain. She asked, "What can I do, Doctor, shall I take herbs, Laetrile, shall I pray?" His answer was "Don't waste your time on all of that stuff, it's all garbage. Just face it and get your affairs in order." The lady went home and killed herself that same day.

Please listen to me when I say that cancer does not mean death. We usually start dying as soon as we hear that word. We have been brainwashed into thinking it's a killing disease and we are supposed to die from it. The doctor may well insist that you believe him when he tells you how much time you have left. No one knows how long you have got—it's largely up to you. If you believe the doctor then you will die right on time. We have seen this on many occasions. Your life is up to you, so don't believe any doctor who condemns you to die just because he doesn't understand your illness. There are thousands of people I have met who were expected to die of cancer years ago. They all had one thing in common, and that is they agreed God is smarter than their doctor.

All I am asking you to do is to change your mind about things, and live. God gave you life, and it's up to you to keep it. Eat properly, think properly, and you will soon notice a difference.

A recent experiment in Europe was very interesting. People with cancer were gathered together, and were all asked this question, "What do you think your cancer looks like, and what do you think of the medicine that you are given to fight it?"

Group A were in accord that their cancer was like a big black rat, very strong and devouring everything, even the medicine.

Group B said that their cancer was a small lump surrounded by white cells (natural immunity), that were gradually eating the cancer away.

Although these people had the same cancer in the same degree, most of group A died and group B lived. Please think about this. Jesus said that faith can move mountains.

Dr. Fernie has another theory on cancer. He claims that cancer patients all fall into a certain category. He explained it to me this way. A woman of 45 has a husband who now devotes all his time to his business. Her children have left home either to get married or to live elsewhere. She develops breast cancer. Suddenly she is at the top of her husband's list so far as attention goes, and the children come rushing home. Could we get cancer just to get our own way? I know that if we concentrate we can eliminate pain, or make ourselves happy or sad. If Dr. Fernie is right and we unconsciously make ourselves ill, then we can just as easily make ourselves well. Faith can move mountains.

At another clinic only a cancer patient who has passed a test as a positive thinker will be accepted. Also, the only visitors allowed in to see the patients are positive thinkers—ones who will spread hope and life and enthusiasm. It seems to work, too.

A clinic in England treats its cancer patients with a steady diet of asparagus tips. This seems to work. Yet another gets good results with massive doses of vitamins A and C, plus six glasses of carrot juice each day.

Another believes that we get cancer because our pancreas is not putting out enough enzymes to eat up the protein in our diet, so they prescribe thirty pancreatic enzymes each day.

One doctor of nutrition has had success fighting cancer with a solution made from poison ivy. One man cured cancer, he assures me, with two teaspoons of gasoline each day!

Another man with lung cancer refused to go into the hospital for the treadmill of death. He said he would not accept the fact that he had cancer, and it went away. Many say that my tea brings such hope to people who have had all hope taken away that they believe they will get well as quickly as I—so they do. Faith can move mountains. As soon as we find out that the medical profession isn't all the answer, and people are living in spite of phony death sentences, then we have to choose among many therapies. It seems that everyone who has beaten cancer writes a book about it, and claims to know the secret and the true answer. I am not one of these. I say that seeing that it's your life you are going to save, then take the best from all of them. None of the things they recommend will hurt you, but leave out the gasoline please, there is an oil shortage.

Let's look at it this way. If there are many types of cancers then there could be many types of natural treatments. You must of course purify your blood first. We are about to take advantage of all the knowledge gained by people who fought for their lives and won. Please remember that most of them were in worse shape than you to begin with. First thing, when that nice little old lady shows

offee, tell her to disappear and take the coffee with her.
er forget the white sugar and cream because you won't be
hose either. Now, if you are in a hospital it may be a little
because everyone knows it is almost impossible to get well
in a hospital. Just be careful of what you eat. Try to get lots of fresh
fruit and vegetables, raw if possible. Whole wheat bread only. Eat
twenty raw almonds each day. Take five pancreatic enzymes before
each meal. Don't eat canned foods, and stay away from salt. Eat
twelve ounces of asparagus each day and, if it must be canned, use
the Jolly Green Giant kind because it has less acid in it. Try to get
lots of fresh carrot juice and drink it within an hour of being made.
Get some Laetrile tablets and take four 500 mg. tablets each day.

I don't want to shock you, but coffee is good for one thing,
and one thing only. That is a coffee enema. You laugh, but thousands
of people do this daily and it's simply wonderful for ridding the body
of toxins and cleaning the liver. Three cups of strong black coffee
in an enema bag, lukewarm. Lie on your right side and try to hold it
for fifteen minutes, then expel. You will soon find out how much you
needed it. You will find it hard to believe all the junk you have been
hanging on to all these years. Please don't worry about this becoming
habit forming. I know of many people who have had coffee enemas
every day for years. As soon as they stop they eliminate naturally
again. At one clinic in France they won't let you stay if you refuse
to have your regular coffee enema. Here you are, already worrying
if it's habit forming, when just now you were sure you were going
to die right away. You see, we've made progress already!

You can drink as much of the herbal tea as you wish. It's
God's natural food so it won't harm you and there are no side effects.
Even the Russian hockey team drinks it daily, just to stay healthy.

One more thing. If you are going to keep on smoking, then
forget about all of the above. Out of the thousands of terminal patients
that I have spoken to during the last three years not one smoker has
survived, and it didn't matter what he tried. Once a heavy smoker

myself, I can hardly stand to be in the same room with someone who is smoking.

You must quit smoking if you want to live, and if you want to live, then you will. Faith can move mountains.

Chapter 7

A NEW LIFE

If you have been subjected to cobalt radiation and/or x-rays then you are suffering a little from radiation poisoning. It's no accident that doctors and nurses disappear behind lead doors while they bombard you with rays.

Here's how to get rid of the ill effects.

Pour one pound of pure salt purchased from a health food store (not iodized) and one pound of baking soda into a hot bath and stay in the water for twenty minutes. Immerse the part affected if possible. Do this twice each week for one month. If you have any surgical scars or radiation burns, spread vitamin E liberally over the affected parts.

Many people I have spoken to have gallstones on top of their other problems. Here is what a top American nutritionist told me to do about this, simply and easily without surgery.

My whole family has done this successfully.

Drink one quart of apple juice daily for five days. This will soften up the stones to such an extent that you can squash them in your fingers.

On the sixth day skip dinner, and at 6 PM take a tablespoonful of Epsom salts with water. Repeat at 8 PM. At 10 PM make a cocktail of four ounces of olive oil and four ounces of fresh-squeezed lemon juice. Shake vigorously and drink right down. In the morning you will pass green stones varying from the size of grains of sand to some as large as your thumb nail. You won't feel a thing, but will be amazed at the results. Thousands have done this successfully.

I would like to say that my heart goes out to you. I don't know you but I know what you are going through. Thousands are going through the same thing as you right now, so you are not alone. You have been luckier than the others for you know that you don't have to die; you can live, as so many of us are doing. You can tell of your recovery and so help others. I didn't start to live until I had cancer, and I know that it will be the same for you. Miracles are happening every day in many places. At the Hans Nieper Clinic in Germany, and the Contreras Clinic in Mexico, just go and see for yourself. You will be surprised. Read the many books all about cancer at your local health food store. Cancer is a mystery only to the medical profession who knows nothing whatsoever about the most important thing in the world, nutrition. Stay away from negative people—you don't need their bad vibrations. Tell them to stay away until you are better. Start planning on how you will be spending next year and the year after. Plan to spread the good word throughout the country. Cancer does not always means death.

Modern-day medicine in North America spends all of its time treating effects instead of causes. They never find out what causes a swelling, but they treat the swelling. If you cut your finger badly, and then let it get dirty, blood poisoning will set in. After a while a red line will travel up your arm and cause a lump under your armpit. The correct way to treat this is to get rid of the poison and also treat the finger, then the lump will disappear.

Right now it's up to you, completely. Think that you are going to live—like Jason Winters and thousands of others. Watch what you eat. Remember that out of seven years of medical training, American doctors have only had six hours on nutrition. You are solely, completely and definitely 100% responsible for yourself. Whatever other people want to do to you, you must always remain captain of your own ship.

In the hospital, you are surrounded by people who think you are going to die because they don't understand cancer. Red-eyed friends and relatives gather around your bed telling you that everything is going to be fine, even though they don't believe it.

You are there with cancer and your mind runs wild. Every little ache and pain says, "My God, it has spread to my right eye, my

38

left shoulder, my big toe." Just because you have cancer does not mean that you are immune from all the everyday aches and pains that everyone has to endure. Ninety-nine times out of one hundred the pain you feel is totally unrelated to cancer. Get that firmly set in your mind. The white cells are eating your cancer, and with a little help from you, the tumor may soon be gone.

Getting well again for you will include purifying your body by freeing it of toxins. Fruit, vegetables, fresh juice and the herbal tea will do this, as long as you are not pouring more poisons into your body at the same time.

You also need an enema regularly. It comes as a great surprise to many people to learn that Jesus spoke to the Essenes about enemas. As a matter of fact, there is a whole sermon that He gave on the subject of healing in *The Gospel of Peace*.

"Seek therefore a large trailing gourd, having a stalk the length of a man; take out its innards and fill it with water from the river which the sun has warmed. Hang it upon the branch of a tree, and kneel upon the ground before the angel of water, and suffer the end of the stalk of the trailing gourd to enter your hinder parts, that the water may flow through all your bowels. Afterwards rest kneeling on the ground before the angel of water and pray to the living God that he will forgive you all your past sins, and pray to the angel of water that he will free your body from every uncleanness and disease. Then let the water run out from your body, that it may carry away from within it all the unclean and evil-smelling things of Satan. And this holy baptizing by the angel of water is: Rebirth unto the new life."

Pick up this book and its sequel, *The Gospel of the Essenes*, and read them carefully. They show that God really does want us all to be healthy—and that is why He gave us instructions that are so explicit. We must pay close attention to this wisdom, remembering that the internal parts of our bodies are perfect places for breeding all types of germs and bacteria, being dark, warm and damp.

Take a positive step; don't think about it, just do it. Buy a bag of fresh fruit. An apple, an orange, a banana and a packet of unblanched almond or apricot kernels. Go for a walk and as you walk, eat the fruit and know that with every bite you are getting enzymes enough to help you. Each step you take will build up your muscles, and the apricot kernels or almonds will give you protein and B17. Already you are doing something sensible to get back to good health. Do this twice a day. You will soon be over the shock and in a better frame of mind. Know with every step you take that another reader in the next town is doing the same thing. We have reports that thousands are doing just this, every day across the country. Now is the time to get into step with this new army of people. They, and you, are following others who have already won the fight.

Please believe me when I say that this could be the most important turning point of your life. You have at last stopped your headlong, selfish rush through life, and now you can stand still for a moment, and look around. Those of you who have not noticed the beauty of the world will certainly do so now. Those who were their own god, ignoring their Father in heaven, will find themselves forced to follow God's wisdom in order to survive, and will love Him for every day He gives them. Be humble, assure Him that you will help others from now on, and if you mean it, you can live a very long happy life. Today, then, is the day you start living. God will bless you.

Chapter 8

THE IMMUNE SYSTEM

The world's leading manufacturer of Laetrile (amygdalin), with head offices in Germany, explains cancer this way:

In spite of numerous costly efforts of medical science, the reason for the uncontrolled division of cancer cells is still unknown. Even a single cell shows a remarkable ability to adapt and survive.

If its environment is disturbed or changed, the cell will immediately adapt itself. This powerful adaptability is comparable to the growing tolerance of insects to pesticides. It is definitely a fact that inflammation or constant stress can lead to cancer. The formation of a cancerous tumor is the defence of the attached cell to survive.

The immune system in our body detects and controls the beginning of inflammation. It gives the order to remove or neutralize damaged or destroyed cells.

But if stress or inflammation continue, for example in skin cancer caused by overexposure to the sun, or in cancer of the stomach and intestines caused by permanent psychological stress, enzymes give orders for cell division in order to bring the body back to its original healthy state.

The natural survival process begins. But the sick cells confuse the immune system by posing as healthy ones. The result is the gradual reduction of constant orders for cell destruction.

This weakened immune system can no longer differentiate between a masked, resistant cancer cell and a healthy one. Therefore an uncontrolled division of sick cells takes place.

The immune system of the cancer patient must be activated to the point where it can once again identify the sick, steadily dividing cancer cells, and kill them. This means that the immune system must be forced into an emergency situation. Many practitioners have been successful by administering megadoses of certain vitamins, vegetable or mineral substances. This brings about an elevation of the immune system where it can once again identify and destroy cancer cells. Unfortunately, unwanted side effects can occur through such overdoses.

Amygdalin/Laetrile/B17 is an extract from bitter almonds or apricot kernels. It is of the utmost importance that only the purest form of this substance be used.

The molecular structure of this substance consists of a cyano group which is very toxic. Only the right, exact procedures in its making will guarantee the ineffectiveness of these toxic substances. Now harmless, the cyan in the Laetrile stimulates an alarm situation in the cancerous body. Our bodies do not only need vitamins and minerals, but also enzymes. It is therefore of the utmost importance that enough enzymes are administered directly to the bloodstream during the phase of activation.

Many alternative therapy clinics are administering an intravenous drip solution of enzymes and Laetrile at the same time. This is most successful. Clinical tests have brought almost instant relief even to long-suffering cancer victims. Also, an insulin-dependent diabetic, for instance, once the pancreas was activated in this manner, showed such progress that insulin injections could be drastically reduced. Rheumatic and gouty pains disappeared.

This information was sent to me for entry in this book. I have visions of bleary-eyed cancer patients asking, "What did all that mean?" It means simply this. If your God-given immune system was working properly, you would not have cancer. We now have to start it working. Laetrile will set off an alarm that will wake up your immune system.

EARLY WARNING SIGNS OF CANCER

After talking to over 10,000 cancer victims we found that in every case they had suffered at least three, and often all, of the following danger signals from three to eighteen months prior to cancer. There are other warnings which the body may provide, so if in doubt, seek medical advice.

1. Weakening of the eyes, necessitating two or three changes of eyeglasses in just a few months.

2. Fatigue. You can never get enough rest. You are as tired when you get up in the morning as when you retired at night. You have little or no energy.

3. Nerves. You become easily agitated and quickly fly into a rage. You hurt the ones you love. Self pity overcomes you and you could easily cry. You become too nervous to go out alone or enter a crowded room.

4. Depression. Life no longer seems worth living. Nothing excites you any more. Morbid thoughts creep into your mind. You quite often become preoccupied with death.

5. A strange tingling, aching sensation deep in your bones. In bed you feel that you must keep changing position, and when you do, the aching only goes away for a few minutes.

6. Loss of interest in sexual intercourse.

Chapter 9

ANXIETY

A well-known psychiatrist said, "In the beginning was the word, and the word was anxiety." This pretty well sums up most people's lives. We worry about the endless varieties of hazards, difficulties and disappointments that lie ahead of us.

From the moment we are born, we are surrounded by uncertainties and insecurities. Murphy's Law tells us that life is tough, that few things work out well, and that if a thing can go wrong it usually will. We find out that our idols have feet of clay, that doctors can be wrong, that our favorite movie star is really quite terrible. We are told that God is dead and there is no one to stop companies from putting poisonous fluoride in our drinking water, or tons of white sugar in baby food.

Fear is something tangible, and we can usually deal with that. But anxiety is a very different matter. Anxiety is a state of mind, and is far more lethal. I say *lethal* because all of these problems eventually manifest themselves in physical illness.

People suffering from anxiety usually do not know which way to turn, so they do nothing. This only increases their anxiety.

Growing up is often one long anxiety. "How is my school work? What about the pimples on my face? What job should I choose? Will I be able to keep it? Will people like me?" Then, a few years later, we fall in love and get married. "Will it last? Will he still love me? Who will change first? Who will die first? Will I be able to cope?"

No wonder we keep getting ill. With anxiety a person becomes inbound, an introvert. Serving others is a surefire way to become mentally well. Keeping busy serving others with kindness and love will usually dispel all your anxieties.

Believing in God is the prime prerequisite because anyone who thinks their life has no meaning, that the world happened by accident, and there is no purpose to anything, has a damn good right to have anxieties.

Tests have shown that most cancer patients suffer from anxiety prior to the appearance of the tumor. My case was no exception. Months before my tumor, I felt nervous, tense and strangely agitated; even walking into a crowded room bothered me. My right tonsil (site of later cancer) would itch constantly. On going to a doctor, he put me on Valium. This depressed the symptoms and allowed the cancer to grow undetected, until it was almost too late.

Tests sometimes show that most people suffering from mental disorders are simply allergic to certain foods or have a total lack of a necessary chemical or vitamin in their body.

Chapter 10

TIBET

Four years later

The ancient Yogi stepped out of his small hut, high in the Himalayas. In spite of the bitterly cold weather and the deep snow, he was clad only in a thin loincloth. His bare feet sank deep into the snow as he made his way to the small field opposite his hut.

He then sat down in the snow, arranged himself in the lotus position, closed his eyes and began to concentrate. In his mind his spine was a white, hot flame, increasing in size and temperature.

The strangers who had gathered to watch were all, without exception, wearing very thick clothing, including heavy parkas with fur hoods. They were still cold.

The old man did not move a muscle, but soon it was evident that he was perspiring. Beads of sweat poured down his forehead, arms and chest.

Whispering started among the bystanders. "Could it be, is it possible?" Yes, it was true. The snow around the Yogi had started to melt and trickle away, only to refreeze once outside a six-foot radius.

Wider and wider became the circle around the man. The snow once four inches deep had now gone, and the bare earth could be seen.

Another fifteen minutes found the Yogi in the center of a circle six feet in diameter and completely devoid of snow. Steam arose from this circle, and from the man.

The Yogi then stood up and returned to his hut.

The bystanders walked over to the circle and, taking off their gloves, felt the bare ground with their hands. The heat was like an oven. It soon cooled, however, and the bystanders continued on their way.

Only two were left standing in the circle. Jan looked up at me from under the hood of her parka, and I returned her gaze. No words were spoken as we turned and walked slowly down the mountain trail to the village of Nangchen.

Learning that there is more to life than just existing, more to life than eating, drinking, breathing and working has brought to my life renewed enthusiasm and vitality.

To find myself standing on a mountain in Tibet, watching the ancient Yogi definitely was exciting, and a far cry from selling refrigerators back in Canada.

It came about this way: One morning, while relaxing in my study in the sixteenth-century cottage that we now call home, on the south coast of England, I received a very strange letter, postmarked Taiwan.

It was from a Buddhist group that had been using the herbal tea for over one year. They were excited about it and invited me to visit with them as their guest. All I had to do was to get there.

My wife was excited about this also, for to get a letter of praise from far-off Taiwan, a country wise in the use of herbs for thousands of years, was praise indeed. I made the journey.

Arriving at the temple tired, hot and out of breath, I was shown to a room with only a table, one chair and a slab of rock on which to sleep. On the table was a pitcher full of water and a bowl to wash in. A drone of male singers echoed through the myriads of rooms and hallways and into my room. As I washed a chill came over me suddenly as I remembered where I was, alone, thousands of miles away from home in an atmosphere so totally foreign to me.

A very old man came into the room carrying a bowl of rice with some kind of vegetable mixed with it, and a bowl of brown drink. I tasted it carefully and behold, it was my herbal tea.

Going into the main hall later that day, I noticed that only men were to be seen, and that these men were all of great age. The eldest was by far the wisest, and although very short and thin, he looked as though he was amazingly healthy. His voice was high and melodic, and he spoke English in flowery tones. He greeted me and shivers ran down my back, and for some unknown reason, the hair on the back of my neck stood on end.

"Did you know, Mr. Jason, that you are 49 years younger than the youngest man at this temple? You are now 51 years of age, are you not?" He smiled at my surprise. "Mr. Jason, I am now 100 years of age."

When I asked him to what he attributed his longevity he answered thus, "You in the Western world are led to believe that you are born, must go to school, graduate, enter college, get a 'good' job, work under high pressure, and at 65 you retire and prepare to die. You have all been brainwashed by very unhealthy teachings from very unhealthy people. You have a complete lack of understanding of life and death. A man does not get wise until he is 65. He has not absorbed everything he can until 80. He is 100 years of age before he can introduce into his daily life this wisdom and experience. He knows instinctively that he is what he thinks, as well as what he eats at this age. The next 40 years of his life are easy and happy. He has no fears of life, death or illness. Apart from an accident, he must remain healthy and productive because he eats and think properly. He has the right attitude toward everything. You in the West expect to die early, so you do. You really make no connection between yourselves and God. Of course, you are a part of God, and with this understanding only then do you realize that you do what you think you will do. Westerners expect to become ill periodically, so they do. They expect to die early, so they do.

"Try expecting to live long and be healthy. Combine this with the wisdom of living and you will do and become whatever you want. Nothing can stop you."

I asked him about the herbal tea and he told me that the monks use it constantly. It's part of the settling of the mind and purifying of the body that we need in order that we may direct our thinking and our lives in the right direction.

I had noticed that the whole time I was there in the monastery that the aged monks would take out a small package of powder and place some on their tongues. At last I ventured to ask about this, and the answer was in one of the most beautiful stories that I have ever heard.

It seems that when Bayan of a Thousand Eyes came out of Mongolia leading his great army, he brought with him hundreds of weak and wounded from continuous battles fought across the continent. After ravaging Peking, they proceeded onto the ancient city of Xian. Once there, the troops were amazed at the number of very old but agile and active people living in that town. They soon found that all the residents of the town took a special herb mixture every day without fail. Babies were fed this soon after they became three months of age. A small pinch of the herbs would be placed on their tongues.

The soldiers also found that this mixture was used only once each day after the morning meal, never at any other time. The local physicians started giving this to the weak and wounded soldiers, who soon found their strength returning very quickly. But something else was happening, too. They also found that they felt better than ever before in their entire lives. Every soldier given this formula, according to legend, recovered. Legend also tells us that they all lived to a ripe old age.

The ancient gentleman leaned towards me and continued, "This herb mixture allows men to enjoy sexual relations over the age of one hundred, and keeps their bodies trim, virile and strong, their minds active and alert. It also allows women to remain beautiful, feminine, and, above all, content into a very old age. That is why we like your formula as much, Mr. Jason, for it is very compatible with what we already are taking, although it serves a different purpose entirely." The formula is called XIAN.

Now we come to Dr. Forbes Ross, who published his revolutionary book in London in 1912.

This man made quite a discovery. To all of his patients he would prescribe 60 grains of citrate of potash in distilled water. He realized even then that people desperately needed potassium to remain healthy. He discovered that in all of his years in practice he never had one patient come down with cancer. Also, the new patients that came to him with cancer were all well soon after taking the potash regularly.

We today suffer from potassium starvation, and it is interesting to note that if cancer is a "germ" disease, it has recently been found that potassium is nature's supreme antiseptic.

Interestingly enough, *The National Inquirer*, March 1983 issue, claims that Karen Carpenter's death was caused by a very low potassium level due to her other problems with anorexia nervosa. I quote, "Low potassium levels cause irregular heartbeats which can lead to heart failure."

Potassium is needed as a daily supplement, so I have added it to the Jason Winters **"Take It For Health"** list that is so popular in Europe.

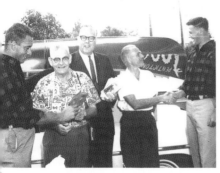

Mackenzie River expedition prep, 1967

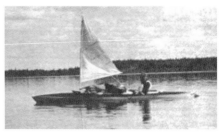

SJW sailing the Mackenzie River, 1967

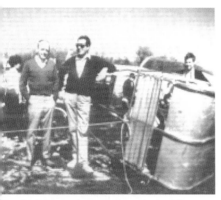

Rocky Mountain crossing - launching
preparations, 1968

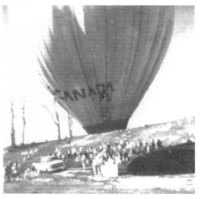

Sir Jason's Hot Air Balloon
"Oh Canada", 1967

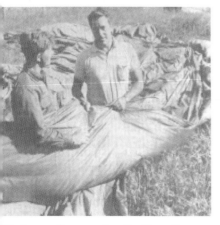

Sir Jason after crossing the Canadian
Rocky Mountains by hot air balloon

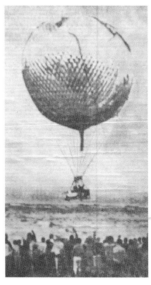

Sir Jason Atlantic Ocean crossing

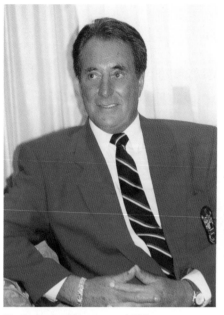

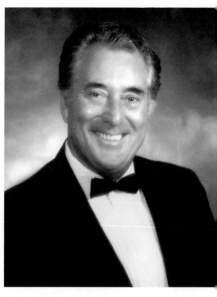

Sir Jason Promo Photo

Sir Jason in Singapore, 1995

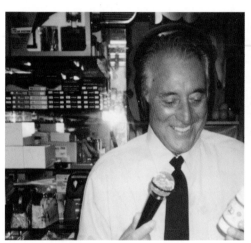

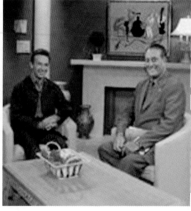

TV Show Australia, 2001
picture by trisun

Radio Show Asia, 1980'S

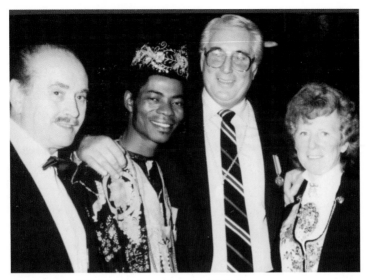

Sir Jason In UK With Prince Obazee, 1980'S

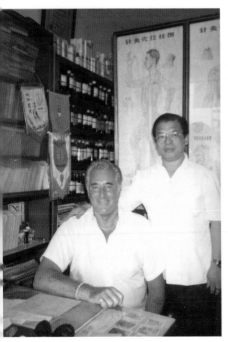

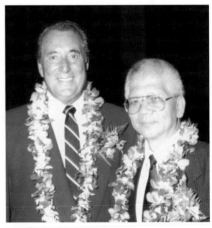

Sir Jason And Steven Soh, Malaysia , 1988

Sir Jason, Hong Kong 1990'S

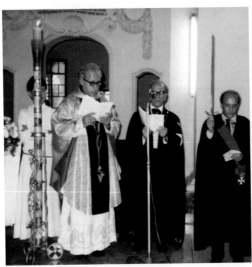

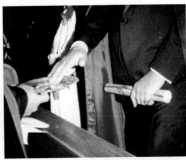

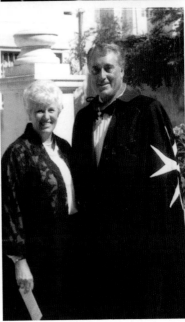

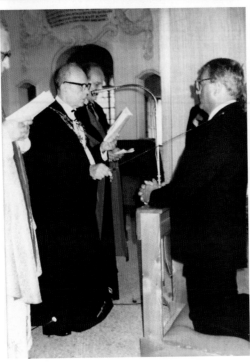

Sir Jason, Knighthood Ceremony, Malta 1985

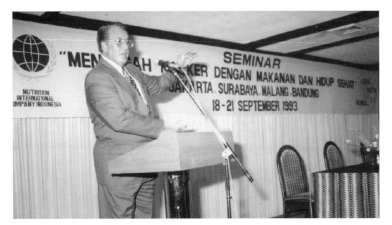

Speaking in Indonesia, 1993

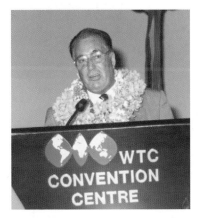

SJW World Trade
Centre Lecture

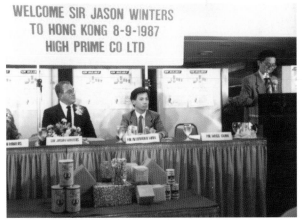

SJW Hong Kong Tour, 1987

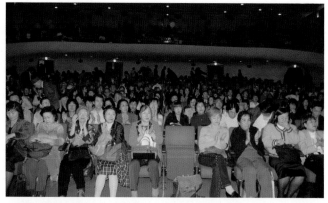

SJW Lecture, Tokyo 2003

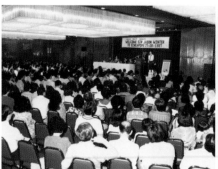

SJW Speaking Engagement,
Singapore 1987

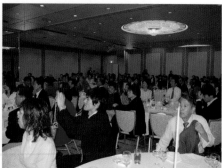

Dinner Gala, Japan 2004

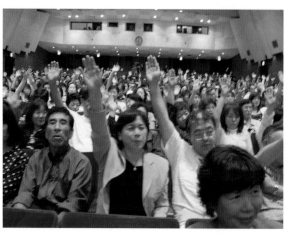

Taking Questions From The Crowd, Osaka Japan 2004

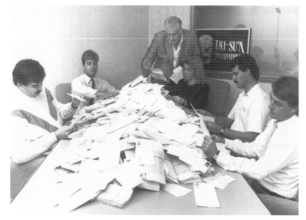

Sorting Testimonial Letters, 1980's

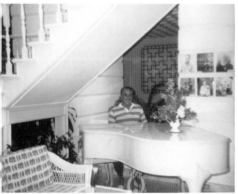

Sir Jason Relaxes Playing Piano, 1990's

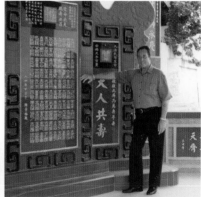

Sir Jason, Hong Kong 2000

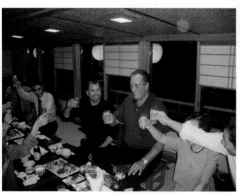

Sir Jason Winters & His Son, Sir Raymond Winters Toasting, Tokyo Harbour 2003

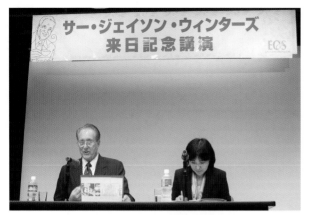

SJW, EOS Convention, Japan 2003

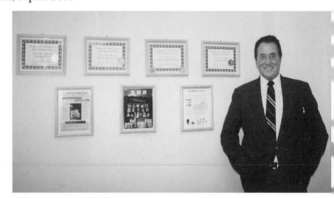

SJW Overseas Office

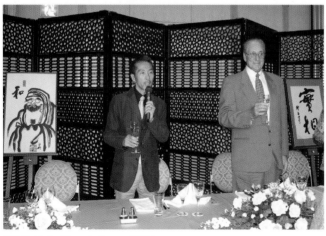

SJW, Gala Event, Japan 2004

Chapter 11

HERBAL LEGACIES

An eagle sat on his perch, high on the mountain, and gazed at the valley below. It was moving as though the whole earth was alive. It was, in reality, buffalo by the millions, all heading south for the winter.

A lone campfire raised smoke down by a small creek, and whenever a buffalo came too close he would be felled by many arrows shot by the Indian braves in hiding. At the same time the squaws and maidens would be gathering herbs and preparing for the evening meal around the campfire. One herb they would pick was well-known for treating swollen joints and fevers, another was for inner strength and well-being. These valuable herbs would be mixed with almost everything the women prepared.

This scene took place centuries before the first Spanish explorer tracked his way across the great American Southwest. Yet the women were well aware that they were practicing preventative medicine and also curing many ills.

There are few eagles left today and hardly any buffalo. The eagle now flies through polluted air, and drinks from heavily polluted rivers. But the knowledge of those ancient Indian women lives on, and it is this knowledge, and not modern science, that will lead the few who will listen through to the new age in good health and safety.

At the same time that the eagle watched the great buffalo migration, another migration was taking place in an unheard-of land half way around the world.

Long before the Chinese were invaded from the north, and long before the cities of Canton and Peking had their first settlers, China was ruled from the capital city of Xian. The migration taking place here was to prove most important to the healers of all China, India and Tibet.

53

Powerful holy men, with a vast knowledge of herbal remedies, would travel far and wide to cities and villages, just for the honor of giving talks in the market places, imparting knowledge to the poor and ailing on how to regain abundant health and happiness.

Some of these travelling teachers found themselves in a far-off high country that would one day be called Tibet. They were excited to find that the rarefied air, due to the extreme elevation, was conducive to clear thinking and spiritual uplifting that allowed them a closer contact with God.

Because of this, many a village would spring up with its own monastery, filled with monks or holy men. Because they believed in reincarnation (many lives) and the law of karma (cause and effect), they were very kind and gentle to each other. Each morning the villagers would lay at the gates of the monasteries baskets of medicinal herbs, which were used by the holy men daily.

Hundreds of years later, in 2838 B.C., the Chinese emperor SHENG NONG would compile the world's first list of these herbs, and their uses. He mentioned 365 herbs in all.

Long before the Mayflower reached America, and long before Ponce de Leon arrived in Florida looking for his fountain of youth, the Viking sailed into natural harbors all up and down the coast of North and South America, from Nova Scotia to Rio.

In South America they found the great rain forests, and were overcome by the extreme dampness, the mildew and the rot that prevailed. Everything was covered with moss, fungus and insects. Everything, that is, except a certain type of tree that stood tall, strong and unblemished. No decay or fungus had touched this tree. No insects made their home in its bark. In this unhealthy climate this tree survived and was every bit as beautiful as the trees they were used to in far-off Norway and Sweden.

The Vikings learned much from the natives of South America, and when at last they were to turn their ships homeward, it was not gold and silver they would be taking back, but bark, bark that would bring a higher price than gold in their own land. For the voyagers had learned that since time immemorial, this bark, made into a liquid, would successfully fight off all diseases and would greatly speed up the healing of accident victims. Medical scientists in South America have recently found that this bark contains a very powerful antibiotic. It is now famous world wide, (except in America) and is proving invaluable to many clinics and hospitals.

It makes no difference what ancient culture we wish to discuss, the fact remains that they knew something that we do not. They were closer to nature and closer to GOD. Their knowledge grew over thousands of years of trial and error, until at last they knew the values of plants and herbs.

Considering the billions of dollars spent by modern science, the results prove that they have failed miserably. But they have succeeded in one respect. They have certainly managed to keep the ancient knowledge written about here a secret in North America, where sickness and medication are the most expensive in the world.

Yet 150 of the world's top prescription medicines come from herbs.

Chapter 12

THE THYMUS

For many years doctors thought that the thymus gland was just something that helped a child grow, and once an adult, then it served no purpose. The thymus lies just beneath the upper breastbone, in the middle of the chest. They thought that once the person became an adult, the gland should shrivel.

As a matter of fact, as recently as the early nineteen fifties, if doctors came across a patient with a large (healthy) thymus they would give him cobalt radiation to try to reduce its size. Many brilliant doctors now know that the thymus is the seat of a person's immune system, and the only reason it grows smaller in most adults in America is because of stress and worry. Dr. John Diamond, in his new book, *Your Body Doesn't Lie*, has proven that you can tell a person's life force through testing the thymus. Beautiful thoughts, paintings and music make the thymus strong; negative thoughts, ugly sights and rock and roll music drastically weaken the thymus and therefore your life force almost instantly.

If you are jealous, vindictive, full of hatred, or closed-minded, your thymus shrivels and you become weak. If a doctor tells you you're terminal, your body will test weak immediately. Just being with a negative person for a little while will leave you feeling weak and exhausted, while the negative person leaves feeling a little stronger.

Dr. Diamond says that he had never seen a sick person who did not have an underactive thymus. He believes that thymus weakness or underactivity is the cause of all illness.

Whether atheists like this or not, while you are in church, or praying, or helping some unfortunate person, your life force strengthens and your thymus becomes healthier.

One thing Diamond mentions is that if you have a group of people in a room, and suddenly someone lights up a smoke, within twenty minutes every person in that room will have the same level of nicotine in their blood. A frightening thought.

In a sad plight in North America are the elderly. They are constantly told by their doctors, "Well, you can expect to be ill at your age," thereby sapping them continually of life force. Add to this the fact that we have been brainwashed into thinking that anyone of seventy years is old, (nothing could be further from the truth) and then the fact that if they do get ill, their whole life savings go immediately to the doctor and hospital, so that even if they recover from this whole negative attitude they have been put under, all they have to look forward to is a meagre old age pension, where they can't even afford the proper nutritious food. As we are all only too aware, junk food is cheap, but nutritious food is almost out of reach for all of us. I wonder if anyone will ever do something about this tragedy. After living in the East I feel that our elderly are dying thirty years before their time, just because they have been told that it is expected. Because of this, I agree with Dr. Mendelsohn, M.D., when he states that hospitals are very dangerous places to go. Not only are they rampant with disease but the negative atmosphere literally destroys the life force of most people, not just the elderly.

After giving the formula of TRIBALENE to an English health food manufacturer I thought I would be free of the health food business. But then I was told about Xian, and I felt that everyone should know about this mixture at once. Both of these products are available freely (but beware of useless imitations).

Xian consists of herbs that will reactivate the thymus, and you have just read how desperately we all need this. Xian is named after the great Chinese capital that was using herbs for healing thousands of years ago.

It is hard to believe that they knew about the thymus, the seat of life, and the life energy so long ago. Xian is destined, I have

58

been assured, to be used widely by all people who wish to remain healthy and in good frame of mind.

Peggy Mason is a spiritual writer living in Tunbridge Wells, England. She is highly psychic and has helped many around the world who just seem out of step with today's world. One of her peeves is cruelty to animals. She claims that we do not get away with anything in this life, especially when we are cruel to defenseless animals. Today for instance, chickens are raised, force fed, in factories specializing in mass production. They are kept all their life in a small cage the same size as their body. No room to move at all, their head is fitted through a small hole in the cage, and they cannot withdraw it, ever! They cannot run, move, scratch or do anything but stand there, all of their lives. This pitiful, desperate, anxious, helpless, unhappy state causes poisons and toxins to course throughout the chicken's body. To eat such a bird simply transfers all that poison to the consumer. And we wonder why we get sick.

Mason also found that unnecessary operations on animals, done simply for practice and fun, have a direct effect on the perpetrator. She was horrified to find at one clinic dogs living in utter terror, because they had been operated on and now had an extra head grafted on. In spite of the absolute cruelty shown them by man, a dog would still look at a stranger visiting and, with head hung low, would try to wag its tail.

Fortunately, these godless experimenters are not happy. According to research, although they somehow can justify this obscene occupation in their own godless minds, they suffer far more illnesses than the average person. Cancer and heart disease strikes them at a far greater rate. That is what is meant by, "As you sow, so shall you reap."

Recently a doctor was so proud of himself while on TV. He explained that weeks before he had forced a white mouse into a tiny test tube and had sealed the end. A tiny hole was in one end so that the mouse could breath. He showed this on TV. The mouse, unable to move backwards or forwards, could only in desperation turn over and over in a futile attempt to escape. The doctor was trying once again to prove that stress causes cancer. This has been proven hundreds of times already!

I was happy to note that the doctor had a serious case of *sanpaku*, which proved that his smiling face belied his true feelings, and could not hide his physical illness.

Now you may think that all this fuss over a mouse or chicken is ridiculous, but I say to you that just because an animal is helpless and can't talk doesn't mean that it has no feelings. It suffers just as much as you would under the same conditions. Participating in this type of experiment, or knowing about it yet doing nothing to stop it, causes a weakening of your life force and will eventually cause the same suffering in your own body to an equal extent.

Cruelty is not conducive to good health. We can't get away with a thing in this life. We don't need a judge and jury to convict us, we do it ourselves. That is what God meant when he said, "Judge not," for we need not judge and sentence others—everyone, no matter how insensitive that person is, sentences himself.

If you are sure you are going to die, then your thymus will shrivel and you will die. If you have faith that you are going to live, then your thymus will expand and start your immune system working at a faster pace, and if you eat nutritiously you will recover.

It is now being learned through extensive experiments that plants can feel. In Canada they found that trees scream when being cut down. They hooked up the trees to a very sensitive hearing device. Hard to believe?

Mushrooms growing unattended in a deserted shed without windows all grew towards the only light available to them, the light shining through a keyhole in the door.

Play beautiful, classical music in a greenhouse and the plants become healthy and strong, and their leaves reach out to the radio, the source of the beautiful music.

Play hard rock constantly and the plants will die in just a few weeks. Their leaves move away from such distasteful sounds. One famous author wrote about such research in his very famous book. He states that every day a man would walk into a greenhouse and shout and curse the plants and flowers. He would call them ugly and tell them they were going to die.

After a few weeks of this, the plants were hooked up to some sensitive equipment. A dozen men walked through the greenhouse, with no reaction, but when the man who had shouted at them entered, all the needles on all of the equipment went crazy, jumping back and forth.

Incredible you say? Would you pay good money to have classical music piped into your cow barn? Many business farmers do because they know they get more milk this way.

Chapter 13

GUIDES TO GOOD HE

The secret of good health lies wrapped with antiquity but it would be wrong to assume the only v. abundant good health comes from ancient times.

The story of GEROVITAL, the "B" complex formula developed by Professor Dr. Ana Asian of Romania, is without doubt tremendously impressive. As a beneficial remedy against the degenerative diseases of old age and maladies of the central nervous system, this product (often shortened to GH3) has a history stretching back 30 years—in more than 70 countries—and an estimated usage by upwards of one hundred million people that cannot possibly be ignored. Bearing in mind the safety and nonaddictive qualities of GH3, it can only be regarded as a most powerful and significant companion to TRIBALENE and XIAN for both remedial and preventative regimes.

America's most famous, most loved psychic, author Ruth Montgomery, writes about Jason Winters and his strange experiences both on the operating room table and after. The book *Threshold To Tomorrow* is causing thousands to write to Sir Jason for more information. The above-mentioned book is now available at bookstores in most countries.

To each of these people he gives the following diet and advice.

JASON WINTERS DIET
Thousands Are Reaping the Benefits of this
Never-Go-Hungry Diet

BREAKFAST

Two Tribalene capsules with a glass of fresh juice. Two slices of whole wheat toast with Fleishmann's margarine. Then take one XIAN capsule.

LUNCH

For lunch, eat a can of Jolly Green Giant asparagus, unheated. Asparagus acid has very beneficial effects on a person recovering from illness.

Take two XIAN capsules after lunch.

SNACK

At three o'clock, have a light snack, a toasted cheese sandwich, while listening to good music. This relaxes you and eliminates stress.

DINNER 7 PM

Take three Tribalene and three pancreatic enzymes thirty minutes before the evening meal. Then eat salad, fish or fowl, brown rice, lima beans, or a soft boiled egg (one), and any fruit or vegetable.

Take one XIAN capsule.

COMPLETE BODY CLEANSE

SKIN

Hot shower, then cold. Dry off vigorously with a rough towel. Your skin will start to come alive and breathe again.

Eat twenty raw unblanched almonds each day for protein.

CELLS

Drink at least three glasses of distilled water daily. This will wash away the inorganic minerals surrounding and suffocating your cells. They will activate and come alive.

MIND

Listen only to good, soothing music. Try to understand poetry. It soothes the mind. Expect the day to be great and it will be. At 5 PM, make a large glass of carrot juice and mix in it two heaping tablespoons of Lewis Laboratory brewer's yeast. Drink it down. It doesn't taste bad and you have just consumed all the vitamin B complex that your body needs. Soon your nerves will be in good shape. That will allow your mind to be restful. Cancer patients should have an additional five glasses of carrot juice daily.

COLON

Healthy people need one soapy water enema each week. Ailing people should have one coffee enema each day and three cups of black coffee, warm. Lie on right side and hold for fifteen minutes. You will be cleansing the liver and colon this way. Coffee causes the liver to exude bile and so cleanse itself. Jason Winters Colon Cleanser also is beneficial.

Keep busy to avoid depression. Join a club, talk to a friend, use your phone.

If you are not working, then GET OUT OF THE HOUSE and go for a walk—for as far as you can, but not more than three miles.

STAY AWAY FROM NEGATIVE PEOPLE AT ALL COSTS. You cannot get well mentally with them draining you.

Cancer patients should take one 500 mg. Laetrile tablet thirty minutes before each meal, after three pancreatic enzymes.

"A recent survey shows that one ounce of whiskey in a glass of hot water is good for everyone (except alcoholics)." Dr. Ian Pearce, *Holistic Approach to Cancer*.

A WORD ABOUT DOCTORS

When I wrote my first book, entitled *Killing Cancer*, I was pretty discouraged about doctors in general. I guess I had the misfortune of having atheistic, uncaring doctors and so had tarred them all with the same brush.

During my hundreds of radio and TV shows, however, I am very pleased to say that I have discovered many dozens of medical men and women who do, in fact, care greatly about their patients. Some have even admitted to me that they pray sincerely for God's help before even attempting an operation.

Many have admitted that nutrition is the most vital treatment in all diseases. Even in the case of accidents, they say proper nutrition is responsible for fast recovery.

INDIA: 1988 JUST OUTSIDE BOMBAY

I was shown a field in which nothing would grow except bitter berries. Once it had flourished with corn and okra. But sacred cattle had wandered into the field and had been slaughtered. Their blood had soaked the ground so that now only bitter fruit will grow that man cannot eat, for it would not leave the body and their juice would stain the very soul.

The field, once valuable, is now worthless. And the owner has moved away.

Chapter 14

WHISPERING WISDOM FROM TIBET

OUTSTANDING QUOTES

"Five billion people in the world, over three billion of them use herbs daily."

Lord Beaverbrook

Hippocrates, the father of medicine, told all student doctors to use herbs for medicine.

Writings from the book *Hippocrates*

The Lord Buddha told the Indian people 2500 years ago that the weak should use herbalene.

Writings of Buddha

Jesus told the Essenes to purify their blood with herbs and all things will fall away.

Gospel of the Essenes

"Doctors and healers must work together toward their mutual goal to heal the sick. Alternative methods of treating illness should not be dismissed as hocus pocus."

Prince Charles

London Daily News 1983

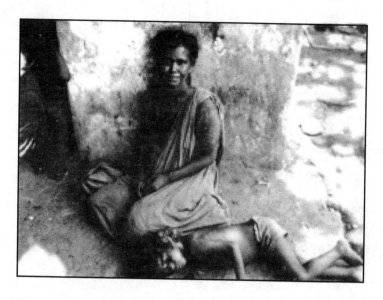

This woman lives here in India with her kids, where she begs for curry and rice.

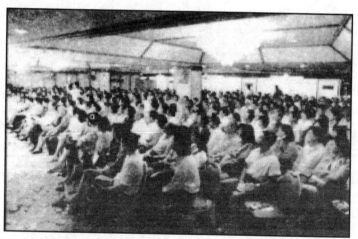

A 1992 Lecture by Sir Jason Winters at the Trade Centre in Singapore to a full capacity audience.

PART TWO

JASON WINTERS XIAN FORMULA

This is a Story of Four

Very Important Things:

1. SELENIUM T

2. GOTU KOLA

3. TIBETAN SPICE

4. YOUR BLOOD

Carefully mixing Selenium T Special Spice and Gotu Kola together for the first time gives us a breakthrough which we call Xian (pronounced *zian*.)

Since arriving in Tibet I have been light-headed. I am not sure whether it is due to the altitude or rather to the great amount of ancient wisdom given to me by my companion. It was from him, a man well over one hundred years of age, that I learned how to eat, think, and be content.

It seemed strange indeed that an ex-terminal cancer patient like me should have to leave America, the scientific leader of the world, and go to far-off Tibet to learn something as simple as how to live.

I could not help thinking that maybe we are the backward ones. I am curious to find out why it is that an old man, living in a small village in Tibet can tell me things that doctors, scientists and highly intelligent men in America are just now discovering, and at a cost of billions of dollars. A person can return from Tibet with specific information on how to prevent and sometimes cure many of man's ills through herbs and diet secrets that have been tried and tested in Tibet for five thousand years.

Some enthusiasts return to America ready to start right in helping people, only to be told a most definite "No" by one agency or another. It seems that a government body must tie up the product for five years and be tested by "one of us."

I am sure that many of us believe that God placed cures for all man's ills right here on earth.

China has 150,000 herbalists who have been making people well for 10,000 years.

Somehow, our medical men are off on a tangent of their own, and could not possibly ask assistance from any other than a medical man with the same training as themselves.

There is no one to tell us how to eat, think, live. Anyone with the knowledge to help is frowned upon and discouraged. We certainly have a long way to go. If you don't think so then try going on a radio talkback show as a guest, and talk about a herb that can help sick people. Every doctor within fifty miles will call in and attack you as if you were the devil himself.

Because of this attitude, many truths are kept hidden. I think one of these truths concerns Selenium T.

The average Tibetan eats a high selenium diet, and they just radiate health. It was because of this that I started looking into the research done on this element in the West. I found that every group of people that has a low intake of Selenium T suffers fatigue, depression, distressing menopause pains, and has more susceptibility to all degenerative diseases, including cancer.

There is a direct relationship between highly civilized countries' processed foods, junk food and lack of selenium.

Selenium is an active mineral that is desperately needed in our bodies, for it is a wonderful antioxidant. It has been shown to prevent or at least slow down the aging process. Also it has become famous in some clinics for slowing down hardening of the arteries. Males appear to need Selenium T even more than women. In the male, 50% of their body's supply concentrates in the testicles and the seminal ducts adjacent to the prostrate gland. Also, much selenium is lost in the semen.

The levels of selenium in the blood of people in various cities has been found to bear a direct relationship to cancer mortality. The higher the levels of selenium, the lower the cancer death rate and vice versa.

FACTS AND ACTUAL TESTS

Because of a report given by Schwarz and Foltz, and encouraged by the same, Hopkins and Maja showed that administration of selenium to children in Jordan with washiorkor stimulated body growth and reticulocyte formation.

Burke reported finding in children from Guatemala with the same ailment, that although they did not respond to a nutritional supplement diet, when selenium was added to the diet, the health of the children improved, and the concentration of selenium in their blood increased to control levels. These finds were confirmed by Levine and Olson.

This means simply that children in Jordan and also in Guatemala that were suffering a disease called washiorkor were cured when selenium was added to their diet. Other diseases also responded when selenium was administered in small doses.

Peridontal disease is a major health problem in New England, a low selenium area.

SUDDEN INFANT DEATH SYNDROME

The studies of researcher Money suggest that sudden death in human infants may result from the combined deficiencies of vitamin E and selenium in cow's milk formulas. During the first month of life, breast-fed infants received more than ten times the vitamin E and more than twice the selenium as infants fed cow's milk formulas.

CARDIOVASCULAR DISEASE

Researcher Frost compared maps of early heart mortality and cardiovascular-related deaths for different areas of the United States and demonstrated an inverse relationship between ambient selenium levels and the death pattern.

Maijanan and Soni, who previously thought that manganese deficiency might underlie the very high cardiac and cancer mortality rate in Finland, have now adopted the view that selenium deficiency, prevalent all over Finland, may be the main contributor.

Lesions of selenium deficiency in rats and sheep have been associated with vascular abnormalities. Demonstrations of the role of selenium in maintenance of membranes may also suggest a function within the vascular system.

CANCER

Investigation of the direct relationship of selenium to human cancer has been limited to demographic studies and to comparisons of levels of selenium in the blood of patients with or without malignancies. Chu and Davidson listed selenium compounds among potential antitumor agents. In addition, Shamberger, and Shamberger et al. associated protection from cocarcinogenesis with antioxidants (vitamin E, selenium, etc.) and food preservation. Harr et al. reported that concentration of dietary selenium delayed or prevented the induction of cancer by N-2-fluorenylacetamide (FAA). The effective concentration of dietary selenium in the torula feed in this experiment was the addition of 100-500 $\mu g/g$ of feed.

On the average, the blood of cancer patients was reported to contain less selenium than the blood of other patients. However, the blood of patients with some forms of cancer showed normal levels of selenium.

Mammary adenocarcinomas induced by FAA in selenium-depleted rats were more invasive than those induced in rats fed selenium supplemented foods.

(From the National Research Council.)

REPRODUCTIVE SYSTEM

When it comes to nutritional deficiencies, it seems to be the reproductive organs that suffer most. It is only fair to say that an excess of certain elements can cause just as much trouble in this area.

Selenium has done much to explain the distribution of this element in the reproductive system. This could mean that selenium has specific roles in the reproduction systems of males, females and developing offspring.

Kar and co-workers, and later others, found that the testicular damage induced by cadmium salts could be prevented by the administration of selenium dioxide.

It is the belief of many researchers that selenium transports cadmium away from vulnerable sites to other locations within the testes where it is innocuous.

Muth, et al. find that administering selenium to pregnant ewes prevents myopathy in developing lambs. This has since been confirmed by many investigators.

It has also been confirmed through research that selenium does, in fact, pass from the pregnant mother to the unborn child.

Although selenium is present in cow's milk, human milk contains selenium in concentrations twice as high.

Because of the large amount of mercury used today by both industry and agriculture, the amount of selenium reaching the fetus might be diminished and thereby bring about a state of selenium deficiency in the child, thus the advantage of breast feeding.

Deficiency in selenium definitely affects the general health. Rats fed a selenium-deficient diet over a few generations showed adverse effects on reproduction.

The female offspring failed to reproduce when mated with normal males. The male offspring had defects in their sperm—it was immotile (incapable of spontaneous movement).

In further studies on piglets from selenium-starved sows, it was shown that lesions appeared first in the connective tissue and capillaries.

Sprinkler found that rats starved of selenium suffered a thickening and degeneration in tissues such as the cardiac muscle, testes and retina. Because of this, researchers Sweeny and Brown concluded that selenium deficiency causes primary damage to the vasculature (blood channels) and also had a bad effect on the membranes.

Selenium was found to be an anti-inflammatory mineral, which resulted in selenium tocopherol treatments for chronic lameness in dogs.

Researcher Money found that over forty species of mammals and birds cannot tolerate selenium deficiency. It is all-important in their lives.

Selenium deficiency became an agricultural problem after World War II because of changes in animal nutrition. To deal with this the Food and Drug Administration approved the use of selenium as a food additive.

Although the importance of selenium in the case of animals is well known, little is known about its role in human beings. Reports from some laboratories indicate that selenium may have anticarcinogenic properties. Also, selenium has been found to have some inhibitory effect on the development of tumors in rodents injected with carcinogens

Selenium is used as an antidandruff preparation and also as an antifungal agent in Tinea versicolor.

Alternative therapy clinics around the world are using selenium in small doses to try to counteract degenerative diseases, and great promise is being shown.

GOTU KOLA

"REVITALIZE YOUR SEX LIFE"

GOTU KOLA
THE SECOND INGREDIENT

Gotu kola has been used in many countries around the world, where they claim benefits such as relieving mental fatigue, age spots, aging, brain problems, lack of energy and endurance, high blood pressure, poor memory, pituitary problems, senility, menopause and loss of vitality.

This herb, mixed with the others mentioned, restores sexual desire and activity within just a few weeks. This approach is natural, with no harmful hormone injections or tablets. Doctors will not give hormones to people with cancer, or to those susceptible to cancer. If ancient Tibetans enjoy sex in their nineties and older, then why should we not be able to do the same?

It seems that Gotu Kola strengthens the mind, gives one the ability to cope with life and its stresses. Many say it gives renewed confidence and zest for life.

Many alternative clinics around the world are using this herb with success. Once carried from India on the backs of mules, this herb is now grown very successfully in Tibet, and is used both in Tibet and India for mental problems of all kinds. Combined with the vital spice from Tibet, we have Xian.

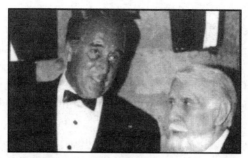

Sir Jason Winters SOSJ (left) seen talking to Count Alberto Carlos at the Italian Ambassador's Ball. Manila 1999.

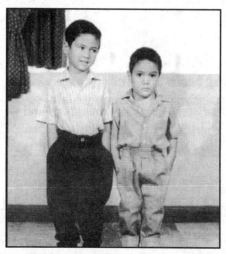

The Golden Lion Children - Jason's sons born while author was in his sixties, thirteen years after he should have died.

SPICE FROM TIBET

Hundreds of years ago, a great army pushed its way across Mongolia, China and Tibet, raping and pillaging every foot of the way. In spite of confiscating all the poor farmers' crops, the soldiers were quite often very hungry and would have perished in the winter blizzards if it were not for the secrets passed down to them for thousands of years. One great secret was SPICE. Not just an ordinary spice, but one to give strength, purity and stamina. At night, while the weary soldiers slept, the "Physicians and Medics," who were really herbalists, would scour the countryside looking for healing herbs.

The spice we call TIBETAN SPICE was really a find, for this particular herb was the one they knew would put all the soldiers who were feeling poorly back into shape quickly.

It seems that even in those days there was such a thing as 'sick call,' which was held early in the morning before starting out on another long day's travel.

The herbalists were highly thought of and were carried all day between two horses. They mostly slept and then at night, with the aid of large flaming torches, they foraged for herbs.

So highly thought of were these herbalist-physicians, that during battle they were kept well to the rear, in both luxury and safety.

Not only was it their job to treat wounds and help the fighting soldiers recover quickly, but they were also charged with keeping the whole army healthy. By this I mean that they had to practice PREVENTIVE MEDICINE. If too many soldiers came down with sickness other than wounds obtained on the battlefield, they would be severely reprimanded.

You see, in those days a physician's main job was to teach the soldiers how to keep well. What a wonderful way to look at the medical profession! To keep people well. To teach them how to eat, think and live correctly.

Even in those days they knew that preventing illness was better than treating it, and so the spice mentioned here was treasured by all. This knowledge has been passed down to us today.

Here is what modern researchers say about this particular SPICE.

"It is helpful if you want to burn the candle at both ends." This miracle medicinal herb from early times reputedly cured a thousand ills and prevented the onslaught of old age. Greek doctors of old regarded this herbal spice as a sacred herb. Dioscorides used it as a remedy for sore throats, snake bite, tuberculosis, kidney troubles, ulcers, arthritis and lack of ambition and drive, among other things.

Properly prepared it does away with decay, is good for the memory, makes a person stronger and prevents spiritual depression. "It makes the life force strong until the end," states another authority This means that there is no degeneration of faculties during old age.

In XIAN, it gives the other two ingredients a definite and powerful boost that cannot be denied. Grown in America, this spice can only be as good as the nutrients in the earth.

If the correct nutrients are missing in the ground, then the herb or vegetable has no good effect on the body. We in America, however, are content with growing food that looks good but in reality has no food value. We also shower the earth with poisons and chemicals to make plants grow quickly and larger than normal. Then, quite often, we polish the food with wax that is definitely detrimental to a person's health.

In actuality we end up eating something that looks great but is an almost "dead food" in our bodies.

Tibetan spice is carefully grown. It is cultivated in naturally rich soil, containing all the ingredients that God intended which are so necessary to our good health.

81

LIFE IS IN THE BLOOD

Every religion and culture has said that life is in the blood. For many years man has known that his blood, and the unrestricted flow of it in pure form through his body, was synonymous with good health.

Blood is, of course, the bearer of life, for it carries oxygen and nutrients to every part of the body, while also removing poisons and gasses.

Vedic beliefs state that the flow of blood is actually the flow of life, for life is in the blood as it courses through our body. Stop the flow of blood to your foot, and it dies quickly, and the same goes for every part of your body.

For the blood also contains forces such as energy which our bodies receive from the sun, the spleen and the heart, changing these solar forces into usable energies which vitalize the body.

How obvious this is today. Give someone a blood transfusion from a sick person, someone for instance who has AIDS, and it will quickly kill the recipient.

The importance of the blood can be seen in the fact that when blood leaves the body, death occurs. When blood stops coursing through our veins, the same thing happens.

During the menstrual cycle, the flow of blood stops long enough to create another life. Ceremonies have been held for thousands of years, idolizing the blood, shedding blood at human and animal sacrifices, smearing blood of freshly killed animals on the body to attract spirit entities that are said to materialize by using the prana, energy of the blood.

The red mineral known as bloodstone has been used in ceremonies dating back 40,000 years and from all regions of the world. Bloodstone is still used today as an antidote to bites, especially snake and other venomous reptiles.

In modern day society blood has been replaced by wines, and is now called "the Blood of Christ." Many peoples of the world believe that the blood controls the body through the soul that is in the blood. For thousands of years man has believed that blood is a kind of liquid fire and some reincarnationists believe that the blood holds a complete record of a spirit's hundred lives. Buddhists practice a system whereby a person can tell all about another human being by the color of that person's heart blood.

Unhappy thoughts make the heart blood the deepest red, almost black. Happy thoughts make the heart blood bright red.

A WORD OF WARNING

Mentioned recently in a New York paper: "More than eighty thousand deaths each year are caused by infection caught while in the hospital."

According to the American College of Obstetricians and Gynecologists, "Up to 90,000 Caesarean sections could be avoided each year, considerably reducing the risk of maternal death, as well as length and cost of hospitalization." (Dr. Robert Cefalo, Committee Chairman, *U.S. News and World Report*, March 22, 1982.)

Not too long ago, a medical doctor in New York stated on television, "over 150,000 unnecessary operations are performed each year in America."

The fight on behalf of Laetrile, Xian, enzymes, DMSO, Chelation, Jason Winter's Tribalene capsules and Freedom of Choice is well known.

Americans are told, for instance, that DMSO is worthless, and yet, in the year 1808, Russian lumberjacks, working in below freezing weather discovered that if they rubbed DMSO (a product of trees) on their aching joints, the pain would quickly leave. Swollen arthritis would also disappear.

THE FOLLOWING WAS PUBLISHED IN *THE BULLETIN*, A
PENNSYLVANIA NEWSPAPER.

"HAS JASON WINTERS REALLY GOT A TREATMENT FOR CANCER?"

In the past few years a lot of attention has been given to one man's extraordinary solution to the terrible dilemma of cancer. His name is Jason Winters and the special capsules which he formulated have been sold worldwide to millions of enthusiastic believers.

The all important question to ask however, is, "Does Tribalene really diminish cancer?" By examining its simple ingredients, we can learn the answer to this ourselves.

Its first and most significant ingredient is, of course, chaparral. Well over a decade ago, this remarkable shrub captured the attention of the medical world for its extraordinary ability to cause tumor regression in some (but not all) forms of cancer. The literature proving this is too abundant to cite for lack of ample space here, but suffice it to say this herb has been more closely looked at for its strong anti-cancer properties than many plants of late have been. A man who has used this herb wrote to me sometime ago of how it benefited him. Mr. Andrew Hanson of Oakland, Calif., testified that chaparral had successfully 'arrested' his leukemia. Another lady from Tempe, Arizona, Mrs. Katharyn Windes, has also contacted me several times about the great value which this shrub has in the management of cancer. In neither case did the parties just mentioned use the word 'cure'; but they did speak about the 'arrest' and proper 'management' of various kinds of malignant cancers in a responsible and truthful way.

One could easily make claims for the Jason Winters' formula in the cure of cancer. I'm quite sure that there are those who would be willing to testify under oath that Tribalene has indeed cured them of one of Nature's most ravaging diseases. But, if you're like me, then you prefer that which is closer to reality. That's why I feel comfortable with the words 'arrest' and 'properly manage' when describing the effects which Jason Winters' Tribalene can have on various kinds of cancer. After all, if it worked for Jason, then why shouldn't it work for someone else, too?

Jason's other common ingredient is red clover. Jethro Kloss, America's greatest herbalist of the twentieth century, continually stressed the use of this fine herb throughout his book and especially in those sections where cancer is specifically mentioned. Of this wonderful herb, Jethro wrote: "Red clover is one of God's greatest blessing to man. I have used red clover blossoms for many years with excellent results. When I was a boy my parents had me gather it for their postmaster who had a serious cancer. He lived to be an old man, without an operation." (*Back To Eden*, p.301).

The final ingredient that makes up the unique Winters' package is a rare herb from Southeast Asia, which Jason has romantically dubbed 'herbaline.' This precious spice not only gives the tea a different flavor but actually enhances the performances of the other two herbs and makes them work better. This synergistic effect is only achieved in the Winters' formula. Other competitors have sought to imitate his formula with blends of their own, but to no real avail. The English, who Jason has officially authorized to manufacture his formula, spend the majority of their time with just his products alone. Unlike their competitors, they can devote a lot of attention to turning out a high-quality product. But when other companies that already carry dozens and dozens of single herbs and combinations get into the act, it's mostly for monetary reasons. Why should they spend a lot of unnecessary manufacturing time for something as special as this, when they've got an entire line of products to worry about? So they just crank out a cheap imitation of the real thing and peddle it along with the rest of their wares.

Unfortunately such unethical practices as this are to be expected in the free enterprise system. This is why Jason and the people who make his products, carry his portrait, signature and *J. W.T.*

on the Winters formula they make. This is to assure buyers of the genuine article and not some phoney reproductions.

When you consider what Tribalene contains, it is no wonder that so many people speak well of it in the health field today. Chaparral has been proven scientifically. And besides that, famous Amish writers such as William McGrath have spoken highly of the herb, too. In his 'Mountaineer Commentary' column of June 27, 1979, in *The Budget*, McGrath not only praises chaparral for cancer but also specifically makes reference to Jason himself.

Thus, while we may refrain from using the definitive word *cure* to describe Jason Winter Tribalene, we can say with all honesty and sincerity that it does 'arrest' and 'manage' various kinds of cancer, not to mention all of the other wonderful health benefits it can also yield.

THE FOLLOWING IS TAKEN FROM THE WRITINGS OF MR. CARL RICHARDS, ENGLAND'S OLDEST LIVING PERSON, 113 YEARS OF AGE:

Looking into Mr. Winters' report on Xian brought back memories of the time I resided in Lhasa, Tibet. I lived there from 1930 to 1938 and learned many of their health habits. Since that time I have consumed daily the substances that Jason Winters has joined together, Gotu kola, Spice and Selenium. I found that they must be taken in exact proportions, which always proved a difficulty, but now, with the advent of Xian, they are both measured correctly and placed in tablet form. I thank Jason Winters for doing something so wonderful, yet so simple. It has been said that the greatest breakthroughs will be the simplest ones, and Xian is no exception. I believe that these ingredients are necessary to maintain life and today so many people are drastically lacking them that they are leading what I call 'half lives.' I am alive today because I visited the Himalayas and Tibet and learned these truths. Now Jason Winters is doing what I should have done forty-five years ago, and that is to make this knowledge available to everyone.

Carl Richards,
London.

It was Bombay, India
September 1988

I was the guest of a talkback radio show that covered quite a large part of India. A man called in to say that his friend was dying and wished to see me. I hastened to tell him that I was not a doctor. He said he knew that, but would I please come to see him.

The caller was in the waiting room just outside the radio room when I left one hour later. We got into the car and he instructed my driver on which way to turn. He was a small, thin man with big bright eyes and he talked constantly.

In ten minutes we arrived at a lean-to made out of cardboard resting against the wall. This is where his friend lived. I crouched down and entered the so-called dwelling. A very old man was lying on a filthy piece of carpet and he was obviously in great pain. I sat next to him and told him my name. He was very excited as he held my hand. It seemed that he knew more about me than I had realized. He suddenly gripped my hand very hard as a searing pain went through him. Knowing what he was feeling, a tear rolled down my cheek. He saw it and said, "Are you crying for me, my son?"

"Yes," I replied. He became furious at me. He told me not to weep for him, or to feel sorry, "for in one million years time, on the farthest planet that you can imagine, you will be walking down a country lane and will see a man walking towards you. When you get close you will look into his eyes and think, 'We have met before.' That is when, my son, we will meet again." With that he died.

All the way back to the hotel I wept, for I had gone there to comfort him, but with his last breath, and in great pain, he comforted me. May God grant that we have such strong faith, regardless of our religious beliefs.

HOPE IS YOUR
MOST VALUABLE ASSET

The medical profession's biggest argument against any alternative therapy is that it gives a patient false hope.

There is no such thing as False Hope. One of the wisdoms learned in Tibet is that words spoken to a sick person are like a weapon. Words spoken by a person's God-like doctor are taken for granted to be true.

How many times have you heard a doctor say, "We've done all we can, the rest is up to the patient. He must have the will to live."

The doctor is saying, in effect, that if the person has the will to live, then their chances are much better. Why is it then, especially in the case of cancer, that doctors send people home with "just three months to live"? Just by saying that they actually cause it to happen. They have taken away all hope, have superseded even Jesus when he said, "Faith can move mountains."

Tibetans believe that if a person has faith and hope, his body manufactures certain chemicals that aid in the curing. But if the patient is convinced that he will die, then his body manufactures chemicals to fulfill his belief.

Every religion in the world says it. *If you want to do something bad enough, nothing can stop you.*

History books are full of people who won out against all odds. Every hero that we have ever heard of did this, and every man, woman, and child is capable of "winning out," regardless of their circumstances.

This is what the book, *The Power of Positive Thinking*, is all about. It's what the Bible is all about. If you have an inferiority complex, you go to a psychiatrist and he tells you over and over again (under hypnosis) that you are as good, if not better than anyone else. Finally you believe it, and so you are cured.

If you constantly tell a child he is stupid, then eventually he believes it and so acts stupid. Encourage the same child every day by saying he is bright and will achieve, and he will.

I believe that when a person is very ill, they hang on to every word their doctor utters. I have seen the excitement that rushes through a person's body when the doctor says, "You're going to be all right."

I have seen the person fall apart and die quickly when the doctor pronounces the death sentence. All of us must be careful of the words spoken to the sick. Jesus says that miracles can happen. So how can we dare, even if we are the most educated and intelligent doctor in the land, to call Jesus a liar and to thereby quicken the death by weeks, months, or maybe years?

THE MIRACLE OF PURE WATER

The sun shines on the sea and lakes, causing vapor to rise and form clouds. This vapor is pure. It leaves behind all bacteria and, what's even more important, inorganic minerals. Inorganic minerals cannot be used by the body. Rain water, travelling over limestone and other minerals in the ground, carries these minerals to plant life. The plants, vegetables, fruit, then use these inorganic minerals for food, changing them into organic minerals. This is when the human body can use them to advantage. These are the minerals necessary for our good health.

Rain water is no longer pure because it has to fall through layers of filthy air, and because distilled water acts as a magnet for toxic materials, by the time it hits land it is also toxic.

Hard water, or any water other than distilled water, is full of lime salts, calcium, magnesium, sodium, iron, copper, silicon, nitrates, chlorides, viruses, bacteria, chemicals, and many other inorganic materials detrimental to the body. Over five billion tons of dissolved minerals are washed into the sea every year. Because of this, sea life has been reduced fifty percent over the last thirty years. Pesticides and factory waste are responsible for most of this.

Many thousands of people are under the false impression that bottled water or filtered water keeps them safe. Treated bottled water does kill the bacteria, but does not remove the minerals that are just as harmful.

If you have a private filter that you use, it still only removes bacteria, leaving the harmful minerals. Plus, some experts say that a filter only works well for the first two days, then turns into a breeding ground for bacteria, thereby defeating its own purpose. Also, experts say treated bottled water is full of dead bacteria, which, although not directly causing illness, does definitely set the groundwork, entering the body and eventually acts as a compost heap or fertilizer for bacteria to grow and spread.

The idea of drinking water was originally to flush poisons from the body, washing every cell daily. Each living cell in our body is a life of its own. It needs to take nourishment from the blood and to expel poisons. Imagine, if you will, that inorganic minerals that you have been consuming since birth in your water supply have surrounded almost every cell of your body, making it impossible for the cell to do its job properly, if at all. This is degeneration, illness, and death, not only to that particular cell, but to you as a person.

Throw drinking water on a glass or mirror, and when it dries you are left with spots. That is the inorganic minerals that are even now surrounding each cell, making it difficult to live a normal healthy life. Take distilled water and do the same. You will find that it leaves no spots at all.

Well water is every bit as harmful, but there is good news at last. Start drinking distilled water, and only distilled water. It makes everything taste better. Also, it acts as a magnet in your body, leaching out all of those harmful minerals that have been accumulating around every cell since the day you were born. It washes every cell and, I think, because of the thousands of testimonies I have read, will do away with aging and most ills. Water distillers are available in many sizes, and we consider ours as the most important appliance in our home, making our lives so vibrant and happy. Try distilled water for one month and you won't believe the results. Xian works well, but with distilled water it is dynamite. Every group in the world known for longevity has access to pure water with no minerals. It truly is a Godsend.

Chapter 15

SPACE AND YOU

Excerpt from a live radio show with Reverend Paul Shaw and Sir Jason Winters.

(Reverend Shaw just finished explaining why there were no such things as UFOs, no outer space beings, nothing but us here on earth.)

Sir Jason, still under hypnosis: "You are on a space ship going up in a straight line. You are travelling at the speed of light. You will be travelling at this speed for twenty million years. At the end of that time, you still will have not gone very far, yet you will have passed thousands of moons, suns, planets, stars.

"Yet you, Reverend Shaw, expect us to believe that God created all of this, then said, 'I am going to ignore all of this. But there is a grain of sand out there, drifting in space. I am just going to concentrate on that.' What great audacity anyone that believes that must have," ended Sir Jason. Neither the Reverend or the moderator knew how to answer that reasoning.

Don't waste your life researching flying saucers and trying to prove that they exist. It is very much like someone devoting his whole life to his bicycle. They are both just common conveyances!

If, after reading this book, you still feel sorry for yourself (which is unlikely), then just think: There are five billion people in the world today; four billion believe in life after death and reincarnation. Since you were born, fifty million people have died each year! 150,000 each day! 6250 each hour!

So, if you think that when you die you will wake up sitting on the right hand of God, just make sure you make room for the other 149,999 who passed away with you!

GREAT BOOKS TO READ

Threshold To Tomorrow
Ruth Montgomery
Putnam Publishers

Ruth Montgomery, Americas most loved psychic author, writes about the "Walk In' of Jason Winters and his strange experiences.

The Essene Gospel Of Peace
Edmond and Bordeaux Szekely

****

The old man squatted in the dust beside me, and as we gazed down the Street of Cages in Bombay, he began to speak. "You see, my son, this life is an illusion—it simply prepares us for the real life in spirit—the eternal, everlasting, ever-conscious life beyond the grave. Without loss of awareness we are there, free, happy and painless, happy in the complete knowledge that life is everlasting."

His sparkling eyes shone from amid a thousand wrinkles, and he whispered, "This great truth is hidden from man for fear he may try to reach the spirit world too soon. He must do his schooling on earth first."

Tears came to my eyes as I realized that I had always known this truth. Deep inside, we all do.

SIR JASON WINTERS

HIS PRODUCTS

AND

THE WORLD FEDERATION

OF

INTEGRATED

MEDICINE

A Special Investigative Report
by
Benjamin Roth Smyth

Including the report to the media
by
Dr. Ian Pierce

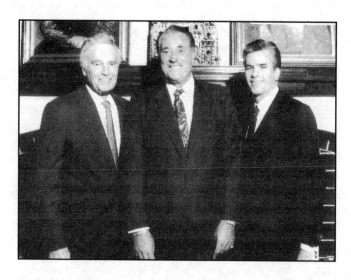

Left to right: actor Charlton Heston, Sir Jason Winters, Congressman John Ensign

Jason Winters discovered Mexican Indian herbs while working on a Hollywood film with Audie Murphy. Here, he posed with one of the Indian "extras" who brewed potent tea from herbs every day on the set.

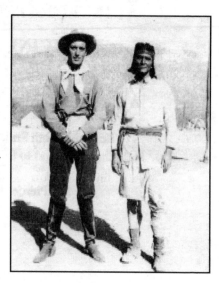

98

The True Story of Sir Jason Winters by
Benjamin Roth Smythe: Scientific Investigator.

London, 1977. The reports of one man's astounding victory over terminal cancer caused great concern and interest. Doctor Ian Pierce proclaimed that Winters had simply found a very potent blood purifier.

I was not to meet the man until the celebration of the British Medical Association's 150th anniversary in London. HRH the Prince of Wales gave a short speech and shortly afterwards I was introduced to Mr. Winters.

He was a quiet man of over six feet tall and around 220 lb. I liked him at first sight. During our conversation 1 realized that this man was nor a health fanatic nor a religious fanatic. He was, in fact, just an ordinary person. His ordeal with cancer was overcome by, in his own words, "fear." He would try anything to get well, even turning to the Bible for help (at the time he was a devout atheist).

The Archbishop of Canterbury helped him pin down the herb referred to in the Bible for blood purification. The writings of Buddha put him in touch with the second herb from India, and his work in Arizona for Universal Studios caused him to locate the third herb used by Native Americans and the Mexican people. Without any knowledge of herbs, nutrition, medicine or faith, he accidently mixed the herbs together and became well very quickly. The rest is history. He discovered no cure but simply something to consume that starts the immune system working.

That was twenty-two years ago. Since that time medical doctors proclaim that Sir Jason Winters has never been ill and looks like he has not aged a day. He looks healthier and younger today than ever before.

Due to Jason's regular radio shows in Tokyo, Bombay, Singapore, Kuala Lumpur, Jakarta and London, his formulas have become the largest selling herbals in the world. His appearance on America's television shows "Sightings" and "Strange Universe" and radio's Voice of America has brought him millions of dedicated followers world wide. I was asked by a motion picture studio to investigate Winters' life thoroughly, to find out if there was a good enough story for a full length movie. And so I went to work.

I started at 21 Stapley Road, Hove, Sussex, England, where Winters was born. His life at that time was filled with sadness and poverty. He had asthma, his father had emphysema and his mother was extremely neurotic. He emigrated to Canada, became a lumberjack, a balloonist, crossed the Rockies by balloon, and canoed the length of the Mackenzie to the Arctic Ocean. He also tried to cross the Atlantic by helium balloon and crashed halfway. He crashed Jaguar cars through brick walls to test safety belts and worked with Audie Murphy and many other top movie stars in western movies.

I was to learn that he smoked forty cigarettes a day, drank half a bottle of whiskey a day and danced in discos until 3 AM. Needless to say he was a hopeless womanizer. I was surprised at first because some of the books written about him portrayed him to be a saint.

I tracked Sir Jason Winters to a small town in India and then on to Macau, China, and from there to the beaches of Fiji. The following month he was in a small town high above the clouds in Malaysia, then as a guest of Suharto in Indonesia.

What an adventurer!

One of the people on the set of the Universal Pictures movie, "Walk the Proud Land", said that Winters had to be half drunk before he could do a good scene.

In 1984 HRH Prince Charles heard that Winters was still alive. Prince Charles was astounded because when they had last met Winters had been just weeks from imminent death. He stated his delight in a letter to Winters. Thus started a friendship between the two men. Because of this and numerous other recoveries, HRH Prince Charles started the Foundation for Integrated Medicine which today is helping hundreds of Englishmen obtain the best of alternative and orthodox medicine.

Dr. Sir Henk Oswald was instructed to visit Winters in America and was so astounded by the sheer volume of letters Winters had received regarding benefits from his products that he nominated Winters for a knighthood. He was flown to Malta for the knighthood ceremony and so he became Sir Jason Winters K.G.S.J. In 1986 he was made Laureate of Belgium, the Netherlands and South Africa. He was given a government grant to finance his search for other valuable herbal formulas worldwide. He has been very successful in this effort. He traces down ancient herbal legends, has the herbs tested by chemical scientists and if they prove valuable, he markets them.

Millions of people use the Jason Winters formulas worldwide. Prime Minister Nikosame of Japan calls Sir Jason Winters Herbal Tea, "quite possibly the healthiest drink in the world." Needless to say, Sir Jason Winters does not smoke anymore and at sixty-eight years of age he certainly does not dance all night, but, when the director of Paramount's television show asked him if he was still a notorious womanizer, he declined to answer.

Sir Jason has since been the guest of kings and princes around the world. He follows the instruction of HRH the Prince of Wales, who told him to "go out into the world and be a peacemaker. Your objective must be to get all of the healing arts to work together for the benefit of mankind. We must get healing to be easily available to all. You must not hate doctors, hospitals, governments, health protection departments, food and drug administrations, for all of them are necessary to combine their efforts to help the sick." Because of his work as the president of the Federation of Integrated Medicine, Sir Jason Winters was given a Certificate of Meritorious service from the United States Congress.

I can not tell you how much I learned and enjoyed investigating Sir Jason Winters and writing the book, *The Sir Jason Winters Story: From Deadly Cancer to Perfect Health*. In my forty years of investigative writing, this story alone has changed my life and has made me feel young again. Yes, there really is hope for us all in this busy and stressful world of today.

I have found Sir Jason Winters to be a simple, unassuming and down to earth person whose objective in life is to tell everyone to have faith, for your darkest day may turn out to be the start of a wonderful life.

BRS

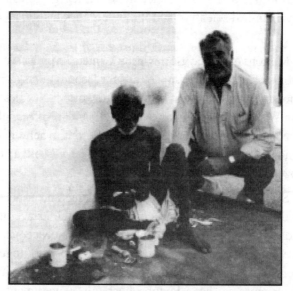

No relatives, No money, No food, No home, No hope.
Bombay, India.
We were able to help.

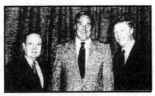

Certificate of Special

Congressional Recognition

Presented to

Sir F.R. Jason Winters

for meritorious achievement

Congressman James H. Bilbray (D-Nevada) together with Congressman Richard A. Gephardt (D-Missouri), are honoring Sir Jason Winters with a Special Congressional Recognition Certificate for meritorious service in creating employment in the U.S. by gaining one million Asian customers.

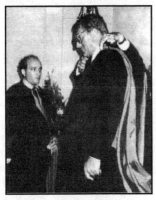

*Sir Jason receiving
Knighthood - Malta*

103

When Sir Jason heard about the foundation that HRH the Prince of Wales was supporting, he thought it was such a wonderful idea that he started the same type of organization for the rest of the world. He is now the President of the Federation of Integrated Medicine.

A very special letter.

Dear Mr. Smythe,

In answer to your request for information on Sir Jason Winters and his activities, I am glad to be of help. He is the only person or company in the natural health field to be given government awards. After twenty-two years in the health field Sir Jason only has twenty products on the market.

The reason for this is that once he was knighted and given a grant to search the world for more valuable herbal combinations, he started in an entirely different manner than other researchers. Because of his limited education in this field, be decided to check out ancient herbs that natives used daily for medicine. He would go to India, for instance, or the Philippines, and often to Malaysia. Once there he would gather the folklore remedies and send them to a laboratory for scientific research, most of the remedies did not work according to the scientists, but of the few out of the hundreds submitted that did work, Winters would try on himself for six months. Only then would he make them available to others. He is only interested in products that he has found to work.

His cooperation with orthodox medicine, medical research, drug companies, government agencies and the Federation of Integrated Medicine has won him awards from not one, but seven, governments. They include Belgium, the Netherlands, South Africa, Malta, Spain, Japan and the United States Congress.

I hope this answers your questions.

Colonel McCauasland
England.

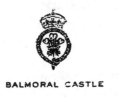

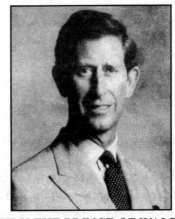

HRH THE PRINCE OF WALES
Patron
Foundation for Integrated Medicine
7th Floor, Windsor House
83 Kingsway, London WC2B 6SD

Dear Sir Jason,

     I felt enormously heartened and touched to read your kind letter recently. How wonderful that you have indeed survived since I last saw you and I am most grateful that you think it may have been something to do with me! I too have been trying my best to bring the orthodox practitioners together with the complementary therapists and after nine years of effort, a bill to regulate osteopathy was passed through Parliament last year as a result. I hope we can now make progress with homeopathy and acupuncture.

     We have also established recently a Foundation for Integrated Medicine with the object of integrating the best of clinical with the best of complementary, or traditional, medicine. We have plans for conducting research projects with various hospital departments in the UK, but we need £3 million to maintain the necessary integrated research. Do you know anyone in the USA who might be interested in helping with the funding?

Sincerely,

Charles

Report to the British Medical Association

Dr. Ian Pierce

A lot of news media attention has been given to a man named Jason Winters and his remarkable recovery from terminal cancer. When I visited him, he was already in good health but grossly underweight. When he was sent home to die after being told that there was nothing more that could be done to help, Mr. Winters turned to herbs and prayer. He contacted Lord Coggan, the Most Reverend and Right Honorable Archbishop of Canterbury. Mr. Winters asked what herb he thought was mentioned in the Bible so many times for blood purification and good health. Lord Coggan did some research and informed Mr. Winters that the herb was quite possibly red clover, which is a herb that has been used in Europe for centuries.

Jason had also heard from a Buddhist monk that Herbalene, an herb from India, was very good for tumors. Also Jason found that the American Indian people use herbs called Chaparral and Sage to cleanse the body.

After obtaining all three of these herbs from three continents, Mr. Winters was making a tea of each one separately which was time consuming as well as ineffective. It was only after mixing the herbs together that the effects of the combination were felt. Mr. Winters' recovery was quite rapid and noticeable.

The news media had a field day with this story. It perked my interest and I finally talked with Mr. Winters. He gave me a sample of the mixed herbs and I had them tested in the laboratory. We found that the herbs are not a cure at all but merely purified the blood to such an extent that a person's natural immune system starts working and the body has a chance to heal itself. These herbs would have the same effect on most illnesses.

The three quality tested herbs are certified organic; they are gentle but a highly effective influence on the body, flushing out accumulated toxins, allowing the body to rebuild cells and return to a healthy state. The herbs are safe and effective with no side effects and work well with other medicines and therapies.

The problem is this, the news media, alternative health people and some religious persons insist on calling the "Jason Winters Herbal Tea" a cure-all, and I must object to this. These herbs do not cure illness, they simply purify the blood and so quite often the body can heal itself. This idea is accepted by most health practitioners and is supported by Mr. Winters.

I have told Mr. Winters on numerous occasions that this is what God intended for all his people.

Dr. I. Pierce, MD

In closing, I would like to add that I stumbled onto a very strange occurrence in my travels while researching material for the *Sir Jason Winters* story. A natural health company in Kuala Lumpur, Malaysia, had so many good reports from the users of Jason Winters Products that they actually published a book of names, photos, addresses and letters of praise about the product.

I discovered the same thing in Indonesia and another in Manila, Philippines. Three separate companies had taken it upon themselves to publish the actual facts about recoveries and complete satisfaction of the consumers of Jason Winters Products.

I want the reader to know that this has never happened with any other natural health product, unless it is paid advertising. This was done at great expense by enthusiastic, happy people who just wanted to spread the good word, mainly, "FINALLY! HERE IS SOMETHING THAT REALLY WORKS. THANK GOD....."

In this day and age of fantastic, amazing, astounding products, that once purchased, do not work, isn't it wonderful to find something that does!!

LIST OF BOOKS THAT MENTION
SIR JASON WINTERS AND/OR THE HERBAL TEA

Threshold to Tomorrow, Ruth Montgomery, Random House

Unlimited Power, Tony Robbins, Fawcett

Prescription for Natural Healing, James & Phyllis Balch, Avery

Helping Yourself with Natural Healing, Lewis Harrison, Prentice

Herbs Fighting Cancer, Romeo Ticson

Cancer Battle Plan, Anne E Frahin, Pinon Press

Integrated Healthcare, Josef De Ubaldo, Rex Publishing Int

More Encounters with the Unknown, Jaime T. Licauco, Anvil

Options, the Alternative Cancer Therapy Book, Richard Walters

The Nuts and Bolts and Greens of a Healthy Back, Dr. Marcia Schmidt, PERQ Publications

I.A.M Unlimited, Inc. CD ROM Reference Guide

Natural Cures They Don't Want You to Know About, Kevin Trudeau, Alliance Publishing Group Inc.

Painless Cancer Cures & Preventions Your Doctor May Not Be Aware Of, Deanna K Loftis, RN BBA, 2005 JADA PRESS

Correspondence

Jason Winters
PO BOX 94075
Las Vegas, NV 89193

www.sirjasonwinters.com

info@sirjasonwinters.com

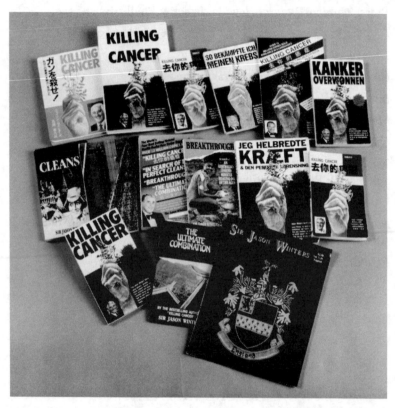

*This book is considered to be one of the most popular books on health
ever written! It has changed the lives of over 12 million people. This
message is so important, it's been printed in 15 languages and has sold
more than 3 million copies in the Mandarin language alone.*

Notes

Notes

Notes

Notes